China's Urban Health Care Reform

China's Urban Health Care Reform

From State Protection to Individual Responsibility

Chack-kie Wong
Vai Io Lo
Kwong-leung Tang

LEXINGTON BOOKS

A division of
ROWMAN & LITTLEFIELD PUBLISHERS, INC.
Lanham • Boulder • New York • Toronto • Oxford

LEXINGTON BOOKS

A division of Rowman & Littlefield Publishers, Inc.
A wholly owned subsidiary of The Rowman & Littlefield Publishing Group, Inc.
4501 Forbes Boulevard, Suite 200
Lanham, MD 20706

PO Box 317
Oxford
OX2 9RU, UK

British Library Cataloguing in Publication Information Available

Library of Congress Cataloging-in-Publication Data

Wong, Chack-kie.
China's urban health care reform : from state protection to individual responsibility / Chack-kie Wong, Vai Io Lo, Kwong-leung Tang.
p. ; cm.
Includes bibliographical references and index.
ISBN 978-0-7391-0660-0

1. Health care reform—China. 2. Urban health—China. 3. Medical care—China. I. Lo, Vai Io. II. Tang, Kwong-Leung. III. Title.
[DNLM: 1. Health Care Reform—China. WA 540 JC6 W872c 2005]
RA395.C53W36 2005
362.1'0425'0951--dc22

2005019739

Printed in the United States of America

∞™ The paper used in this publication meets the minimum requirements of American National Standard for Information Sciences—Permanence of Paper for Printed Library Materials, ANSI/NISO Z39.48–1992.

Contents

Illustrations

Map

Tables

Preface

This book examines health care reform in urban China. This is a topic of great interest and significance to academics, policy makers, and the general public. Not only does this topic concern the well-being of Chinese urbanites, but also China's health care reform experiences should be relevant to other less developed and transitional economies in terms of striking a balance between meeting people's health care needs and promoting economic growth. It is clear that, according to our study, economic growth is not automatically followed by health care development. A strategy with priority in economic growth, as in the case of China, does not bring forth cost efficiency and equity in health care for the whole nation. Nevertheless, we find instances of success in the reformed urban health care system. We do not stop short at problem analysis; one of the aims of this book is to offer theory-informed choices on health care development. We hope that this book will fuel the interest in this area.

We would like to thank Professors Gung-wu Wang and John Wong of the East Asian Institute, National University of Singapore, with which we had affiliations and where the idea of a book on China's health care reform was initiated. We are most grateful to Qin-ying Ci and her post-graduate students for assisting us in the field research in Wuhan, China. We must also thank the Social Science and Education Panel of the Chinese University of Hong Kong for funding our study. Thanks also go to Kit Lam for providing essential research support; Sen Gong for his critical comments; Ching-fong Wong, Xun Liao, and Li-dun Tu for their assistance in arranging the field visits in Shenzhen; and Haicilla Mak, Frances Yu, Kwan-siu Chan, Mabel Yeung, Ching-man Lam, and Vivian Lou for their prompt and timely proofreading assistance. The anonymous reviewer's valuable comments are much appreciated. Finally, we have to thank the staff at Rowman & Littlefield and Lexington Books for their careful production of this book.

Hong Kong and Japan
September 2004

Chack-kie Wong
Vai Io Lo
Kwong-leung Tang

Chapter 1

Introduction

"Health is a sector that cannot simply be left to market forces"

In a feature article, *The Economist*, a pro-market international magazine, advised the Chinese government on health care. It said that China is going too far on privatization and is "beginning to discover that market forces alone cannot produce good health care."[1] It then goes on to suggest that the Chinese, all 1.3 billion of them, live on the coast if they want to have health care that is as good as that in many Western countries.[2] *The Economist* is not alone in taking a critical look at China's health care. A regional magazine, *Asia Times*, is also watching China closely but from another perspective—it suggests that China has lagged behind in health care and that this situation offers investment opportunities for regional powers. A CEO of an Indian health care organization is quoted as saying that "this is where India can step in," because "China is ahead of India in many things but behind us in healthcare."[3]

The most categorical remark on China's health care comes from the World Bank, a supranational proponent of free markets and minimal state intervention. In a 1997 report on financing health care in China, it commented that China faced deep problems in its health sector. The lesson for China was, "Health is a sector that cannot simply be left to market forces."[4] This critical remark was made by the World Bank some years ago, but the message remains relevant. As recently as early 2004, in the wake of the outbreak of the Severe Acute Respiratory Syndrome (SARS) epidemic, the representative of the World Health Organization (WHO) in Beijing, China's capital, said, "Chinese officials are starting to realize that the market alone can't do it on health."[5] Apparently, SARS has taught the Chinese government a good lesson on the role of the state and the division of responsibilities between the state and the market in the provision of public goods such as health care.

These remarks seem to indicate a general consensus on the indispensable role of the state in public health and basic health care protection, a position with which even the main proponents of pro-market policies like *The Economist* and the World Bank would agree. This consensus comes as no surprise as empirical evidence also reveals that the economic miracle of the Chinese economy, i.e., an annual growth rate of 9.7 percent over the past twenty years,[6] has not gone hand in hand with corresponding development in the area of health care. But the most unflattering verdict on China's health care performance comes from a WHO report in 2000. It rates China's overall health care system performance at 144, and fairness of financial contributions at 188, out of 191 member states (see chapter 6). This is alarming—not only because of China's admirable achievements in the economic sphere over the reform era but also because China was once so widely praised for its achievements in raising the standard of health care for the entire population when the country was relatively poor, under the leadership of Chairman Mao.[7]

Nowadays China is wealthier—its GDP per capita (at current prices) passed the US$1,000 threshold for a low-middle-income country in 2003. From the Chinese traditional perspective, this advance already indicates a living standard that equates to *xiaokang*—a moderately well-off society.[8] China's new leaders have already set the target at US$3,000 by 2020 as the next economic development goal.[9] In spite of China's newfound wealth and the pledge of a new economic vision for the nation, the road ahead looks dim in terms of better health care for its entire population. Large disparities in access to health care and in the outcomes of health indicators are found between the coastal and the inner and western provinces, between the urban and rural population, and between the rich and poor.[10] It is fair to say that China still performs relatively well in terms of the health level of its people—it is given a much higher ranking in the above-mentioned report in this aspect (see chapter 6). However, according to the assessment of a think tank in the State Council—the executive branch of the People's Republic of China—the relatively high levels of health are largely a result of past performance, a legacy of the 1980s.[11]

All in all, this brief discussion places health care in China in perspective—economic growth does not automatically bring development in the sphere of health; apparently, the development of policies and systems is tremendously important. In recent years, health care reform has received top priority in many countries, both developed and developing. Meeting health needs is now a daunting task. The Chinese experience, demonstrating as it does the link between health care and economic development, is also relevant to other less developed and transitional economies, many of which are still struggling to find a way to meet the dual goals of satisfying health care needs and developing their national economies.

Health Care Reform in the Wider Context of China's Development Strategy

The earlier strategy, developed by the late Patriarch Deng Xiao-ping, of placing a premium on economic growth may have contributed to the poor performance and the inequity of the health care system in China. The growth-first strategy has also resulted in many of the social problems, such as widening income inequalities and regional disparities, new urban poverty, and rising unemployment, that China is now facing. There are signs of new thinking on China's development strategy under the new party chairman Hu Jin-tao (胡锦涛). Hu recently pledged to devote attention to the "Five Coordinations" (五个统筹) in China's future development—that is, the coordination between urban and rural development, between development of various regions, between economic and social development, between human beings and nature, and between the need for internal development and the demands of opening to the outside world.[12]

Apparently, better coordination between urban and rural development, regional development, and economic and social development has important implications for the future development of China's health care system. In the meantime, there may not be any drastic change of policy on health care. The reason for this is clear: The reformed urban health care system has been in place only since 1998. In the normal course of events, its impact must be fully felt before any drastic change is made in policy or system design. Of course, this speculation is based on the assumption that the Chinese leaders will follow the prevalent incremental approach for reforming its social security system.[13] Perhaps the SARS outbreaks have reminded China that its health care system, especially in its rural sector, is at great risk and in need of a redirection. As an official of the WHO in China has said, a crucial shift in thinking is now taking place due to the outbreaks of SARS, avian influenza, and HIV.[14]

Consequently, there are grounds for believing that a shift in thinking on the policy and system design of health care is about to take place. But how far this change will result in material changes depends to a great extent on whether the reformed urban health care system achieves what the policy makers want and whether it fulfills the health care needs of the ordinary people. On the rural side, a new cooperative health care system is still in its pilot stage, despite the demise of the traditional rural health care system. It is estimated that only 6.5 percent of the rural population was covered by cooperative health care in the late 1990s, compared to 90 percent of villagers in 1976, before economic reform was initiated.[15] There has not been a substantial increase in health care protection for peasants in the past few years. According to the national health care survey performed in 1998, 87.44 percent of the financing sources of health care in the rural areas came from self-payment.[16] No wonder the "return to poverty"(返贫现象) due to illness has risen at such phenomenal rates in rural China. For instance, a report on this phenomenon in Jiangsu Province (江苏省) found that 70 percent of those on state poverty relief benefits were forced to claim these benefits due to illness.[17]

In this work, we confine ourselves to the reformed urban health care system—the reform of health insurance, the reform of medical establishments, and the reform of medicine production and circulation system—because, unlike the rural system, it has already gone beyond the experimental, pilot stage and is now at the stage of full national implementation. Nearly all urban areas are now covered by the new health care system (see chapter 3). Other aspects of China's urban health care system such as health services delivery are generally left out. However, it is worth devoting a little space to the latest developments on the rural side. In 2003, the central government finally took a decisive step by requesting two to three counties in each province, autonomous region, and municipality directly under the central government, to act as test sites for the new cooperative health care for rural peasants. A tripartite financing scheme is proposed, in which the central government, the local government, and the enrolled peasant each pay at least 10 yuan (8.28 yuan = US$1) annually for the peasant to join the new cooperative health care scheme, which funds large medical and hospitalization expenses (see chapter 2). Apparently, the Chinese government is, at last, beginning to take concrete action to address the less developed areas in its health care system. This perhaps indicates a shift in thinking in China's overall development strategy.

Urban Health Care Reform in Focus and the Future Toward Which It Aims

Against this background, the outcome of urban health care reform seems to be critical for China's future health development. As we said before, unlike rural health care, which is in its pilot stage, China's reformed health care system has been in full national implementation since 1998, with a similar overall framework across all cities, although there are differences in the particulars of the various schemes (see chapter 3). In other words, it is now possible to investigate the impact of the new system with empirical evidence taken from a period of moderate duration. On this empirical ground, this book has also a moderate aim—to focus on the assessment of the initial impact of China's urban health care reform. In this respect, it is able to present the most updated empirical evidence on the initial impact of the recent Chinese reforms in health care.[18] Along with the latest government statistics, the findings of two social surveys and three focus group interviews of respondents in Wuhan, a mid-China city, conducted respectively in December 2003 and January 2004, were also available for analysis (see chapters 5 and 6). They allow us to take an in-depth look at the views and opinions of ordinary citizens, medical personnel, and officials in relation to health care reform.

The other aim of this book is to provide a set of choices on health care, informed by the most recent theory. Social policy is about "what is and what might be"; thus, it becomes involved in choices in the ordering of social change.[19] Four influential theoretical perspectives on social policy are examined—state welfarism, neo-liberalism, welfare pluralism, and social developmentalism (see chapter 4). These are normative theories, which seek not only to explain but also to give direction and guidelines for action that will lead to certain desired results. They seek to answer the question, what is good for society? In other words, we do not content ourselves with the "what is," the present conditions, but look for clues for change in terms of "what might be." It is in this regard that normative theories are helpful.

Welfarism played the dominant role in the Maoist era, when people regarded health care protection as an entitlement on the basis of their employment status, and the provision of health care protection was seen as the state's sole responsibility. With the advent of economic reform, this welfarist orientation was deliberately attacked as the underlying cause of China's underdevelopment, responsible both for the poor state of the national economy and the low incentivization and low productivity of state-owned enterprise workers. Economic reform aimed to change this, and especially to change the welfarist mind-set of state-owned enterprise employees. Thus, the reform leaders aimed at a less interventionist state for China. In theory, neo-liberalism does not sit comfortably with socialism, the proclaimed ideology of the ruling Chinese Communist Party. In practice, however, some of the neo-liberal market principles have been adopted in China, as we have documented in the previous quotes from commentators outside China, who believe that the underlying cause of China's present disappointing health care performance is too many market forces at work.

We also present two other normative theories—welfare pluralism and social developmentalism—in reference to health care development. Welfare pluralism is particularly relevant to the present health care context in China because the state now assumes only a minor role among the sources of finance for health care (see chapter 6). This situation may not be desirable, and many have argued that "health is a sector that cannot simply be left to market forces." But the reality of a minimal role for the state in financing health care indicates a larger space for other welfare sectors in an emerging welfare mix in health care arrangements.

If China is really shifting its thinking about its health care system, and of its financing in particular, the normative theory of social developmentalism should be relevant (see chapters 4 and 7). It is compatible with the new leadership's "Five Coordinations" development strategy, the coordination between economic and social development, regional development, and, in particular, rural and urban development. The new development strategy has to be matched with policy structures in practice, especially in finance. However, in 2001, according to official statistics, the central government financed only 6.5 percent of the total public health care expenditure; local governments shouldered the rest[20] Consequently, social and regional disparities were enormous. Against this seemingly undesirable background of an uneven social development in health care, social developmentalism offers an option: harmonizing the need for economic growth and the need for health care. Of course, another vision about "what might be" is the choice in the ordering of social change in health care, and it is pretty much in line with the new development strategy as proclaimed by China's new leadership.

All in all, the four normative theories offer a series of visions against which we can carry out a critical analysis of the reality—the "what is" of the problems in China's health care system—and project the "what might be" for its future development.

Plan of the Book

This book, which is the first book in English on China's urban health care reform, is a systematic study of health insurance reform based on the most recent empirical data from fieldwork in Wuhan. The three authors of this book come from two disciplines—comparative social policy and law. They are all Chinese scholars who have received their academic training abroad but who are very familiar with the culture and language of China and have good connections there. In other words, they do not have the difficulty experienced by many non-Chinese writers, who have to immerse themselves in a language and culture that is foreign to them. Their good connections in China enabled them to undertake the fieldwork needed to collect firsthand empirical data from surveys and interviews. They use a comparative policy framework, supported by the legal expert's knowledge of regulatory specifications, to provide an up-to-date and empirically based critical account of the full national implementation of China's urban health care reform. The focus of the analysis is the Basic Health Insurance, the cornerstone of the emerging urban health care system. Of course, they do not lose sight of the other two components of the new reform package—the reform of medical establishments and the reform of the medicine production and circulation system—both of which are closely related to Basic Health Insurance.

Following the introductory chapter, chapter 2 provides a succinct account of the major features and problems of the traditional health care system as well as the three basic components of the reformed health care system. Attention is also paid to the role played by legislation in policy changes in China. It is important to note that while China has a powerful central government in Beijing, local governments and the local offices of relevant ministries are allowed to enact local statutes to suit local circumstances.

Chapter 3 focuses on the three local health insurance schemes—the Three-Phase Passage Model, the Combined Boards Model, and the Three-Fund Management Model—based mostly on local statutes and specifying the detailed arrangements for local implementation. These local health insurance schemes implement, with variations, the general framework of a socially pooled fund and personal medical accounts in combination. The three major schemes were developed by local governments prior to the promulgation of the 1998 Decree by the State Council on Basic Health Insurance. In other words, the Chinese approach to reforming its health care system is essentially an incremental and bottom-up approach. Chapter 3 also provides an initial assessment of the successes and challenges of health care reform, primarily based on the earlier implementation of the three major local schemes. These pave the way for a critical assessment, in chapters 5 and 6, based on the new sets of data, particularly from the fieldwork in Wuhan, a mid-China city.

Chapter 4 outlines four major theoretical approaches to health care provision—welfarism, neo-liberalism, welfare pluralism, and social developmentalism. We have already briefly covered the rationale for including a theoretical chapter on these approaches. We should not lose sight of the equally important issues "on the ground," such as the fiscal, economic, political, and institutional factors that come into play in the development of new policy. Having said that, however, normative theories have a powerful impact on policy change as well, because they offer broad visions of what the "Good Society" should look like.[21]

Chapter 5 provides a cross-sectional examination of health care reform in China, taking a mid-China city, Wuhan, as a case study. Two medium-scale social surveys were conducted on patients and employees in late 2003 to collect their views on the reformed health care system in their city. In general, it is found that most of the respondents were supportive of the major components of the reformed health care system. They endorsed the policy and ideological shifts. However, they also exhibited support of welfarism, implying that they still endorse the old ethos in which the state is responsible for providing basic health care protection. More important, the respondents were also very worried about the affordability of health care. A complex response pattern is identified, which is compatible with the findings in the literature on public opinions in relation to social policy—people identify strongly with symbolic political beliefs and ideologies on general issues but are much more critical when they come to matters affecting their self-interest.

Chapter 6 asks whether health care reform and the full implementation of Basic Health Insurance have advanced equity in the system. It presents the findings of three focus group interviews—with the patients, the insured workers, and the insurance center administrators. The discursive interview findings are supplemented by the latest available statistical data, including some comparative international figures, so that the subjective views are placed in the wider context for an objective but critical assessment of the initial impact of the full national implementation. It is found that, simply in terms of financial equity and overall system performance, the emerging urban health care system is not an unqualified success story. Indeed, it is in need of redirection. This is not to say that the new health care system has not achieved anything—it is supported by a good budget, which indicates its sustainability in the longer term, and there might have been some improvements in horizontal and vertical equity. In general, the successes of the reformed health care system have been apparent on the cost efficiency side. Placing these successes in the wider context of national health costs and looking at international comparisons, the new system does not perform well at all.

Chapter 7 reviews both the strengths and weaknesses of the urban health care reform, using both previous literature and the results of our study in Wuhan. Taking the criteria of coverage, choice, portability, and cost control, we believe that the current medical insurance program fares better than the old system. However, some weaknesses have emerged, and some of these problems (dwindling government financing in health care, presence of a significant number of marginalized uninsured individuals, heavy financial burdens, etc.) need to be attended to urgently. It is argued that the present health care system is pluralistic; the central government seems to have a strong preference for including other actors in the reform initiatives (including the community, the for-profit sector, NGOs, families, etc.). But such an approach is problematic. It is argued here that social developmentalism should form a central policy framework for China. The central government should go down the route of social development to ensure that social policies and programs contribute positively to development, without creating conditions of welfare dependency or harming economic growth. In this regard, China should build on the country's tradition of intervention to urge policy makers to actively address social concerns like health care needs.

Notes

1. *The Economist,* Special Report: China's Health Care, 21 August 2004, 20–22.
2. *Ibid.*
3. Hua Yan, "China Debates Medical Reform Privatization," *Asia Times Online*, www.atimes.com/atimes/China/FH11Ad04.html, (accessed 26 August 2004).
4. World Bank, *Financing Health Care: Issues and Options for China,* China 2020 Series (Washington D.C.: World Bank, 1997), 2.
5. Jonathan Watts, "China's Shift in HIV/AIDS Policy Marks Turnaround on Health," *The Lancet* 363, no. 9418 (April 2004): 1370–1371.
6. *The Economist.* (21 August 2004), 21.
7. World Health Organization, *Evaluation of the Strategy for Health for All by the Year 2000: Seventh Report on the World Health Situation*, (Geneva: WHO, Regional Office for the West Pacific, 1987); 1–2.
8. *China Information News*, "*Xiaokang*: People are Searching for a Hundred Methods," 4 December 2002, www.people.com.cn/ (accessed 4 August 2003); *China Information News,* National Statistical Bureau Forecast: Three-fourths of People Enter *Xiaokang* This Year End, 23 November 2003, www.people.com.cn, (accessed 4 August 2003).
9. The Chinese Communist Party, "*The Resolution of the 3rd Plenary of the 16th Party Congress*," 14 October 2003, www.people.com.cn, (accessed 14 October 2003); also on a report by the Development Center of the State Council, "The Comparison of China with Countries at US$3,000 GDP per capita," www.drcnet.com.cn, (accessed 4 May 2004).
10. Sen Gong, "China's Financial Health Input and the Analysis of its Performance since Economic Reform," (Internal report no.2, Social Development Department, Development Research Center, State Council, August, 2004) (in Chinese); Shao-gang

Wang, "The Crisis and Change of the Chinese Public Health," *Comparative Studies* (July 2003): 52–88.

11. Gong, (2004).

12. The Chinese Communist Party, (14 October 2003).

13. Chack-kie Wong, "Reforming China's State Socialist Workfare System: A Cautionary and Incremental Approach," *Issues and Studies* 35, no.5 (September/October 1999): 169–194.

14. Watts, (2004).

15. Social Policy Research Center, China Academy of Social Science. *An Overview of Rural Health Care Protection*, (Unpublished report, March 2003).

16. Ministry of Health, *An Analysis Report of the Second National Health Survey, 1998. http://1998.www.moh.gov.cn/statistics/ronhs98/ronhus4/.doc* (accessed 4 May 2004).

17. Social Policy Research Center, (2003).

18. For instance, see Bao-gang Guo, "Transforming China's Urban Health System," *Asian Survey* 43, no. 2 (March/April 2003): 385–403. It should be one of the most recent papers on China's urban health care system, but it still relied on previous data.

19. Richard Titmuss, *Social Policy* (London: Unwin Hyman, 1974), 30.

20. Gong, (2004).

21. Gosta Esping-Andersen, et al., *Why We Need A New Welfare State* (Thousand Oaks, CA: Sage Publications, 2002).

Chapter 2

Health Care in China

Over the years, China has adopted two major systems of health care. The first one, currently referred to as the traditional health care system (传统职工医疗保险制度), was implemented from the 1950s to the mid-1990s. The second one, commonly known as the reformed health care system (职工医疗制度), was launched in the late-1990s and is being actively implemented. These two systems, however, apply only to urbanites because rural residents receive health care under a different system. In that sense, China has a bifurcated health care system, namely, the urban and rural subsystems. Since the present study focuses on health care for urban workers, this chapter discusses the traditional and reformed health care systems in detail but provides a succinct account of rural health care.

The Traditional Health Care System

Prior to the introduction of economic reforms in the late 1970s, China had a command economy. Under such an economy, China adopted an employment-based welfare system to provide its citizens with various benefits, such as old-age pensions, housing, medical care, maternity care, and workers' compensation. Specifically, health care was administered through two insurance schemes—the labor insurance health system (劳保医疗制度) for enterprise staff and workers and the publicly funded health system (公費医疗制度) for personnel of government organs and institutions. The particulars of these two insurance schemes are summarized next.

The Labor Insurance Health System

In 1951, the Government Administration Council promulgated the Labor Insurance Regulations (the Regulations) to provide guidance regarding the welfare benefits of staff and workers employed by enterprises.[1] Although some provisions of the Regulations were subsequently amended by the promulgation of decrees and circulars, the framework outlined therein remained intact. The following discussion, therefore, will highlight the major provisions on health care for staff and workers.

First of all, the Regulations covered (1) enterprises employing 100 or more workers; (2) enterprises in the post, railway, water or air transport industries; (3) capital construction units of factories, mines, and transport enterprises; and (4) state-owned construction enterprises. Enterprises not covered by the Regulations might settle matters relating to labor insurance through collective agreements after consultation between the owners or management of such enterprises and the trade unions. The labor insurance health system provided enterprise staff and workers and their immediate families with insurance coverage for work-related and nonwork-related illnesses, injuries, and disabilities. In respect of nonwork-related illnesses and injuries, the following procedure and benefits were applicable.

When a worker became sick or sustained a nonwork-related injury, he or she should visit the enterprise-run clinic or hospital or a commissioned hospital. The enterprise was to bear the costs for diagnosis, treatment, surgery, hospitalization, and general medicines, while the worker was to pay the expenditure on costly medicines, meals, and fares. Even so, if the worker experienced financial difficulties, the enterprise might provide further subsidies. If the immediate family of the worker became ill, the sick relative might also consult the doctor at the enterprise-run clinic or hospital or a commissioned hospital free of charge, and the enterprise would pay one-half of any cost for surgery and general medicines. Even so, the worker must pay, on behalf of the relative, the cost on expensive medicines, hospitalization, meals, and transportation.

Furthermore, when the worker could not work due to illness or nonwork-related injury for less than six consecutive months, he or she would be paid 60 to 100 percent of his or her normal wages, depending on the length of service. If the worker could not work for six or more consecutive months, the enterprise must provide a monthly sum, which ranged from 40 to 60 percent of his or her normal wages, until he or she could resume work or was pronounced disabled or dead. In fact, if the worker became disabled or had completely lost the ability to work after illness or a nonwork-related injury, the enterprise must provide relief money, which was 50 percent of his or her wages if he or she needed a caretaker, or 40 percent of his or her wages if he or she did not need a caretaker, until he or she regained the ability to work or died. This relief money, however, would not be given to a worker who had lost part of the ability to work but could still work.

In 1966, the Ministry of Labor and the All China Federation of Trade Unions issued the Circular on Several Questions regarding the Improvement of the Labor Insurance Health System for Staff and Workers,[2] which increased the amount of medical payment made by workers. From then on, the worker had to pay fees for registration and home visit. Although the enterprise was to pay the expenses on costly medicines, the worker must bear the cost for nutrients and tonics. When the immediate family of the worker received medical care, the worker not only had to bear one-half of the cost for surgery and medicines but must also pay the fees for registration, examination, and laboratory tests.

As a rule, the worker might first pay the expenses to be borne by the enterprise and then seek reimbursement. Alternatively, the enterprise might directly settle accounts with the hospital. At the beginning, the labor insurance health system was financed completely by the enterprise administration[3] Since 1953, the enterprise drew 5 to 7 percent of its total wages to finance health care, depending on the nature of the industry.[4] In 1969, the Ministry of Finance required the enterprise to draw 2.5 percent of its total wages as welfare funds, 3 percent as bonus funds, and 5.5 percent as medical funds, a total of 11 percent as "staff-and-worker welfare funds."[5] If 11 percent was not enough to cover all medical and welfare bills, the enterprise might draw funds from after-tax profits to make up for the deficiency.[6] These welfare funds were treated as part of the operating cost and managed by the trade union.

The Publicly Funded Health System

In 1952, the Government Administration Council promulgated the Directive regarding the Implementation of Publicly Funded Health Care and Prevention for Personnel of the People's Governments, Parties, Organizations, and Institutions at Various Levels, and the Ministry of Health issued the Measures for the Implementation of Publicly Funded Medicine and Prevention for State Personnel.[7] These statutory provisions applied to (1) public servants employed by the people's governments, parties, organizations (such as trade unions, youth leagues, and women's leagues), and institutions engaged in cultural, educational, health, and economic-construction activities at various levels and (2) disabled military personnel.

Under this system, the government organ, organization, or institution paid the expenses for diagnosis, treatment, surgery, hospitalization, and medicines, while the insured must bear the cost for meals and fares. If the insured had financial difficulties, the government organ, organization, or institution might provide further subsidies and obtain reimbursement as administrative expenses. Thus, the benefits were similar to those provided under the labor insurance health system. In terms of finance, the publicly funded health system implemented by government organs was funded by allocations from the treasuries at various levels, while institutions that practiced differential financial management (差额预算管理) and "self-receipt and self-expenditure" financial management (自收自支预算管理) must establish health care funds.[8]

Medical Establishments and Medicines

For years, the government determined the annual budgets of hospitals, set the wages of hospital personnel, and fixed the prices for drugs and medical services.[9] Since 1980, the government's funding to hospitals had declined,[10] and hospitals began to practice "budget control" management, which required hospitals to keep revenues and expenditures in balance.[11] However, since China's traditional method of cost accounting was based on material costs alone, even though the overall cost of medical services consisted of materials and labor of medical personnel, medical fees based on such a cost accounting method were usually lower than the actual costs.[12] Meanwhile, the gap between the prices of medical services and other prices gradually expanded, and enterprises facing financial difficulties were in arrears with their medical bills.[13] Because the government was unable to provide significant subsidies, its medical pricing policy intentionally allowed hospitals to be compensated through profits from the sale of medicines.[14] That is, hospitals were allowed to receive 15 percent of the differential between wholesale and retail prices of medicines.[15] Moreover, doctors might deduct a percentage of the fee for an examination that required the use of high-end medical equipment.[16] Thus, profits from filling prescriptions and operating high-end medical equipment constituted a significant portion of hospitals' revenues.

Rural Health Care

The labor protection health system and publicly funded health system did not apply to rural residents. In the countryside, health care was administered through the cooperative health care system (合作医疗制度). This system was spontaneously launched by local farmers in the mid-1950s and subsequently affirmed by the central government.[17] Under this system, a health care fund was set up with contributions from members of a production team (生产大队) or commune (公社) as well as subsidies directly provided by the production team or commune.[18] Members received medical treatment or prescriptions free or at reduced price.[19] In 1976, about 90 percent of the rural residents in the country had enrolled in the cooperative health care system.[20]

Problems of the Traditional Health Care System

Under the traditional health care system, workers were provided with a relatively decent level of health care, including free diagnosis and treatment, general medicines, and surgery. In a command economy, this system guaranteed the majority of urban and rural residents basic health care, thereby fostering social stability and economic development.[21] As a result of the decollectivization of the rural economy, decentralization of decision making, introduction of management accountability, and emergence of the private sector, problems of the traditional health care system began to surface.

First, both health care providers and medical service users lost control, resulting in high medical costs, low efficiency, and tremendous waste[22] It has been estimated that unreasonable medical fees constituted about 20 to 30 percent of total medical costs.[23] Apparently, the cause of this problem was two-fold. On the demand side, since medical expenses were largely borne by the employer, employees lacked the motivation to save on medical expenses.[24] Moreover, since only half of the expenses on general medicines for family members could be reimbursed, many patients requested excessive amounts of medicines to share with family members who had not consulted the doctor.[25] On the supply side, since hospitals relied on profits from the use of high-end medical equipment and the sale of medicines to defray operating expenses,[26] many of them over-prescribed medicines or ordered unnecessary diagnostic tests to increase incomes[27]

Moreover, the broad range of medical benefits at little or no cost to workers drained enterprises and the government treasuries.[28] For example, the total medical costs for workers in 1978 was 2.7 billion yuan, but the figure reached 77.4 billion yuan in 1997. During this period, medical costs increased twenty-eight times, but the fiscal income of the government increased only by 6.6 times.[29] Moreover, in 1997, the average outpatient medical cost was 61.6 yuan, and the average inpatient medical expenditure was 2,384.3 yuan. Compared with the figures in 1989, outpatient medical expenditures increased at the average rate of 26 percent, and hospitalization expenditure increased at the average rate of 23.8 percent, which were higher than the average increase rate of the general price index during the same period.[30] Thus, the treasuries at various levels as well as enterprises or institutions found it difficult to bear the financial burden.[31]

Despite the enormous medical cost, the coverage of health care under the traditional system was relatively narrow because only urban workers in institutions, state-owned enterprises, and some collectively owned enterprises were able to obtain free or cheap medical services.[32] Hence, although foreign investment enterprises and private enterprises had developed rapidly, workers in those enterprises were not able to enjoy their lawful right to basic health care.[33] Indeed, since health care was tied to employment and there was a discrepancy in the level of medical services received by workers employed by various enterprises, the resulting low labor mobility in turn slowed down the development of a labor market.[34]

Furthermore, enterprises did not have any rational mechanisms, and thus, steady financial sources, to pool funds to pay the medical expenses of their workers.[35] When enterprises experienced financial difficulties, they either contracted a low volume of health care or were in arrears with reimbursements for medical fees.[36] Therefore, many workers did not receive the basic health care to which they were entitled.[37] In other words, the capacity of the labor insurance health system to resist risk was low.[38]

As a result, medical services under the traditional health care system were rendered as social welfare. In this way, the traditional health care system imposed a heavy financial burden on enterprises and the state treasury; resulted in high medical costs; benefited only certain segments of society; hindered labor mobility; and had a low capacity for risk. With the intensification of economic reforms, these problems made it difficult for the traditional health care system to sustain itself. In addition, the decollectivization of the rural economy resulted in the disintegration of rural communes, which, in turn, made the continuous functioning of the cooperative health care system infeasible. To improve the quality and efficiency of health care, intensify social security reforms, and facilitate the reform of state-owned enterprises, the Chinese government has launched three reform programs: the introduction of a health insurance scheme covering the basic medical needs of urban workers, the reform of medical establishments, and the reform of the medicine production and circulation system.

The Reformed Health Care System

Starting from the 1980s, enterprises and local authorities began to undertake measures to reform the health care system.[39] For example, workers were required to bear part of their medical costs, normally 10 to 20 percent, with an upper limit set for self-payment. A contract responsibility system (定额包干) was introduced, in which enterprises provided health care providers with a year-round budget for taking care of a certain number of employees.[40] In 1988, the State Council approved the formation of a research group on health care reform headed by the Ministry of Health.[41] The research group drafted a proposal, which recommended that medical costs be borne jointly by the employer and the employee, and four cities—namely, Dandon, Siping, Huangshi, and Zhuzhou—should be chosen as the test sites.[42] In 1989, some municipalities began to set up social pooling schemes to cover the medical cost of retirees, while others launched pooling schemes for serious illnesses.[43] Nevertheless, these measures were undertaken within the framework of the traditional health care system.[44]

In 1993, the Third Plenary Session of the Fourteenth Congress of the Chinese Community Party decided on a health care system combining a socially pooled fund and personal medical accounts (统账结合).[45] In the following year, the State Council approved the selection of two medium-sized cities—Zhenjiang in the Jiangsu Province and Jiujiang in the Jiangxi Province—as the test sites for implementing this policy. The State Commission for Structural Reforms, Ministry of Finance, Ministry of Labor, and Ministry of Health also jointly promulgated the Opinion concerning Test Sites for the Reform of the Health Care System for Staff and Workers.[46] Based on this opinion, Zhenjiang and Jiujiang formulated their respective implementation plans.

The health insurance schemes of Zhenjiang and Jiujiang were successful,[47] and valuable lessons could be drawn from their experiences. On 8 April 1996, a national conference on the Basic Health Insurance was held. Participants from all over the country were instructed to formulate health insurance plans for their respective areas and publicize and educate citizens about the importance of health care reform. The State Commission for Structural Reforms, Ministry of Finance, Ministry of Labor, and Ministry of Health jointly issued the Opinion concerning the Expansion of Test Sites for the Reform of the Health Care System for Staff and Workers.[48] Based on this opinion, over fifty cities became the test sites of health care reform.[49]

In December 1998, the State Council promulgated a landmark decree, the Decision concerning the Establishment of the Basic Health Insurance System for Urban Staff and Workers (the 1998 Decree).[50] Thus, in 1999, the labor insurance health system and publicly funded health system were unified into the Basic Health Insurance System for Urban Staff and Workers (城镇职工基本医疗保险制度). The underlying objective of the health care reform is to provide better-quality medical services at relatively cheap cost in order to satisfy the basic medical needs of the masses.[51] As mentioned earlier, the current health care reform consists of three major components: the introduction of a health insurance scheme covering the basic medical needs of urban workers, the reform of medical establishments, and the reform of the medicine production and circulation system.

The Basic Health Insurance

According to the 1998 Decree, the Basic Health Insurance is to be established in all types of enterprises, institutions, and government organs nationwide. In addition, the Basic Health Insurance must be managed under the unified leadership of the local government (属地管理). Although health insurance schemes may vary in accordance with local circumstances, the general framework of the Basic Health Insurance is composed of a socially pooled fund and personal medical accounts. Both the employer and the employee must pay insurance premiums. All the money in the socially pooled funds and personal medical accounts must be used for paying medical expenses (专款专用).

Under the Basic Health Insurance scheme, workers go to designated health care providers (定点医疗机构) for diagnosis and treatment. Thereafter, they can fill prescriptions at the hospital's outpatient pharmacy or at designated drug retailers. Designated health care providers are certified by the Ministry of Labor and Social Security and must sign contracts with the social-security-administration organ in order to provide medical services. Insurance subscribers can change health care providers either upward or downward in terms of the level of medical services. Moreover, the social-security-administration organ is supposed to manage the socially pooled fund and personal medical accounts.

To implement the 1998 Decree, the Ministry of Labor and Social Security, Ministry of Health, Chinese Medicines Management Bureau, and Medicines Supervision and Management Bureau subsequently issued accompanying rules, such as the Provisional Measures on the Administration of Designated Health Care Providers under the Basic Health Insurance for Urban Staff and Workers,[52] the Provisional Measures on the Administration of Designated Drug Retailers under the Basic Health Insurance for Urban Staff and Workers,[53] the State Catalog of Medicines for the Basic Health Insurance,[54] and the Opinion on the Administration of Diagnosis and Treatment Items under the Basic Health Insurance for Urban Staff and Workers.[55]

Because the Basic Health Insurance is meant to cover all urban workers[56] and to ensure that the level and mode of health insurance matches the country's level of productivity and the capacity of various parties concerned,[57] its slogan is "low level, broad coverage."[58] As a matter of fact, the primary objectives of the Basic Health Insurance are to transfer the administration of health care from individual employers to local governments—the socialization of health care administration— and to make the government, enterprises, and workers share the cost of health care.[59] In particular, the establishment of a socially pooled fund is to promote mutual aid, while personal medical accounts are designed to encourage people to save for future medical needs and to control waste resulting from excessive medical expenses.[60] To ensure both fairness and efficiency and to bring into play the initiative of workers, what a worker can enjoy under health insurance should match his or her contribution to society.[61]

Notwithstanding the Basic Health Insurance, an enterprise or government organ may provide supplemental insurance, especially for workers who used to enjoy more comprehensive medical services or who are suffering from or will have serious illnesses. If the employer provides supplemental health insurance, the maintenance costs can be paid out of the worker welfare fund, if it does not exceed 4 percent of the total wages. If payment out of the worker welfare fund is insufficient, the employer can, after obtaining government approval, treat the excess as part of its operating cost. Furthermore, workers can subscribe to commercial insurance provided by outside companies if they want high-level medical services. For poor people who are unemployed or patients who have used up all the funds from available insurance channels, medical relief is the last resort. Thus, the Chinese system of health insurance is pluralistic and multilayered. It is pluralistic because several sources together fund the overall health insurance scheme, namely, government, enterprise, worker, and donation. It is multilayered because the means of payment for medical costs consist of various levels: individual savings (personal medical account and personal funds), family assistance (supplemental), a socially pooled fund under unified collection and management (mutual aid), enterprise insurance (supplemental), commercial insurance (supplemental), and medical relief (for people in poverty).

There are two major reasons for a pluralistic and multilayered health insurance scheme. First, since the socially pooled fund covers only the basic medical services, there is plenty of room for developing other types of insurance due to differences in income level and medical needs.[62] For example, in Shanghai, the average medical consumption rate per person in 1999 was more than 17 percent of the total wages.[63] Since the social health insurance covered about 8 percent, it was necessary to develop other insurance channels, such as enterprise supplemental insurance, for the payment of the remaining 9 percent.[64] Second, it is recommended that regions, industries, and enterprises that used to provide medical services above the basic level establish multilayered health insurance, thereby guaranteeing the connection of the new and old systems as well as the steady implementation of medical reform.[65]

In 1994, there were about 3.75 million workers and 257,000 retirees participating in the Basic Health Insurance; by the end of 2002, about 69.26 million workers and 24.75 million retirees had subscribed to the Basic Health Insurance[66] (also see Table 6.1). The increasing number of subscribers demonstrates that the implementation of the Basic Health Insurance has gained full momentum. To provide more details about the implementation of the Basic Health Insurance, chapter 3 will discuss various local practices.

Reform of Medical Establishments

According to the 1998 Decree, local authorities should establish a system to separately manage and account for the provision of medical services and the provision of medicines (医药分开核算，分别管理的制度), formulate competitive mechanisms for medical services and medicine circulation, rationally control the level of drug expenses, strengthen the internal management of medical establishments and drug stores, regulate the behavior of those providing medical services, decrease personnel and increase efficiency, reduce the cost of medicines, and normalize the prices of medical services. In separating the provision of medical services from the provision of drugs, local authorities should also lower the proportion of income from filling prescriptions to the total income of a medical establishment, raise the quality of medical personnel and medical services, actively develop community health services (社区卫生服务), and incorporate the services of community health centers into the coverage of the Basic Health Insurance. In this connection, the Ministry of Health and relevant ministries and departments should formulate plans for the reform of medical establishments and policies for the development of community health services.

Consequently, in 2000, the State Council Office for Structural Reforms, State Planning Commission, State Economic and Trade Commission, Ministry of Finance, Ministry of Labor and Social Security, Ministry of Health, Medicines Supervision and Management Bureau, and Chinese Medicines Management Bureau jointly issued the Guiding Opinion concerning the Reform of the Urban Health and Medicine System (the Guiding Opinion).[67] This directive lists various structural reforms that the government will undertake to reform medical establishments as well as the medicine production and circulation system. The following discussion, therefore, will highlight the major provisions.

First, health care is to be administered as an industry. That is, the administrative-subordinate relationship (行政隶属关系) between the Ministry of Health and hospitals is to be abolished, with the former serving the supervisory role and the latter serving the technical-service role. Formerly, the Ministry of Health managed hospitals (办医); from now on, the Ministry of Health supervises medical establishments only at the industry level (管医). Moreover, a new system of "managing medical establishments by category" (分类管理) is to be established. Under such a system, medical establishments will be classified into profit-seeking and not-for-profit establishments. There must be separate fiscal, tax, and pricing policies for profit-seeking and not-for-profit medical establishments, and the latter should receive preferential tax treatment. Specifically, if a not-for-profit medical establishment is run by the government, the prices of its services should be set after government subsidies and income from selling drugs are subtracted from the cost. For other types of not-for-profit medical establishments, the prices of their medical services should follow the price guidelines issued by the government. Profit-seeking medical establishments, however, may autonomously determine the prices of their medical services and must pay tax in accordance with the law.

Similarly, a service system of community health centers, general hospitals, and special hospitals should be established. The community health center should focus on preventive medicine, health maintenance, health education, birth control, common illnesses, and the treatment of and recovery from chronic illnesses. General and special hospitals should focus on the treatment of diseases, especially acute, serious, and complicated illnesses. Even so, transfer between medical establishments must be provided. At the same time, enterprise-run clinics located in the city should be transferred gradually to the local government for the purpose of achieving unified management. In fact, conversion, cooperation, merger, and grouping of hospitals are encouraged to secure the rational distribution and utilization of medical resources. Furthermore, to rectify the problem of having hospitals supported by the sale of drugs, the provision of medical services and the provision of medicines as well as their respective incomes and expenditures are to be managed separately. For instance, outpatient pharmacies at hospitals should be converted into independent drug retailers.

As a result of the reform and resulting competition, the management level of hospital leadership, the doctors' consciousness regarding medical expenses, and the quality of hospital services have improved.[68] Moreover, hospitals have either streamlined their operations or merged with others to remain competitive. For example, in Shanghai, hospitals have formed groups to provide more efficient medical services in accordance with the principle of "large ones leading the small ones" (以大带小).[69] Ruijin Hospital concentrates on complicated diseases, Luwanqu Center Hospital treats patients for common diseases, and Shizheng Hospital is used for recuperation.[70] Nonetheless, enterprise-run clinics were not put on the list of designated hospitals because they did not have sufficient computer capacity or due to certain perceptions about their leaders, which caused inconvenience to workers because they had to take leave in order to consult doctors and their wages and bonuses were deducted.[71] Indeed, as long as the balance of revenue and expenditure of the health insurance funds was maintained, local authorities would not exert too much control over hospitals.[72] Currently, there is the mistaken belief that "the law will not punish the masses" (法不责众) and that hospitals have been required to refund only for their violations of regulations.[73]

More important, an increasing number of hospitals have entered the market. For example, in March 2004, the government of the Xinxiang City of Henan Province signed an agreement with the China Huayuan Life Industrial Company of the Huayuan Group to establish a hospital management company, to which the private company contributed cash and the government contributed the hospitals' net assets. The private group owned 70 percent of the equity, while the government owned 30 percent. This management company would manage five hospitals in the city, and the term of agreement was fifty years.[74] Similarly, in 2003, the Suqian City of Jiangsu Province, through auction and transfer agreements, made all the public hospitals in the city privately invested (民投), privately owned (民有), privately managed (民办), and privately operated (民营). This move had generated criticisms from various sectors of the society and caused the concern of the Ministry of Health. However, one official of the Suqian City defended that the move was a reform measure, namely, converting the "management of health by government" (政府办卫生)into the "management of health by society" (社会办卫生).[75]

In view of this wave of privatization of hospitals, one scholar and the representative of a hospital association had respectively expressed the following concerns: In the past, the government managed public hospitals by means of administrative measures (行政管理方式). Although hospitals have entered into the market, the government is not prepared to play its supervisory role, especially in terms of quality, price, and safety requirements. In particular, the government has not yet outlined its policies in a document that can provide guidance on how to reform medical establishments, for example, what types of hospitals should be kept and how many hospitals should remain public. Thus, although local authorities have adopted various means to implement reforms, some public hospitals have been trying to expand. The government should uniformly manage medical resources. Moreover, since the reform of hospitals has been conducted mostly through the selling of equity or cooperation, the different objectives of public hospitals (not-for-profit) and private hospitals (profit-seeking) will inevitably result in conflicts. Furthermore, hospitals are institutions, but a framework of reforming institutions has not yet been established. It is inappropriate to apply the measures for reforming state-owned enterprises to reform medical establishments because institutions and enterprises are different. Last, the acquisition of hospitals by business groups also raises antimonopoly concerns.[76]

Reform of the Medicine Production and Circulation System

As previously mentioned, the State Catalog of Medicines for the Basic Health Insurance has been issued for the implementation of the Basic Health Insurance. The Guiding Opinion states that the prices of the medicines listed in the catalog are to be set in accordance with government directives, or alternatively, the government will determine prices for these medicines. The same will apply to preventive drugs and necessary children's medicines. Indeed, the government may draw up uniform retail prices nationwide. For other types of medicines, drug manufacturers will set their prices in accordance with the price regulations of the state. To regulate the behavior of medical establishments in purchasing medicines, the government will promote centralized solicitations of bids. Furthermore, the retail price of a medicine will be printed on its packaging gradually, but invoices based on the actual price of a medicine must be produced at every stage of sale.

To prevent the repeated formation of low-level pharmacies and to ensure the production of quality drugs, the Guiding Opinion instructs the government to draw up rigorous entry requirements for drug manufacturers. In fact, based on the types of medicines, drug manufacturers must meet the requirements under the Standards regarding the Management of Production Quality of Pharmaceutical Manufacturers (abbreviated as GMP in English) by various deadlines. To ensure the safety of medicines, the government will strengthen its supervision over drug wholesalers and retailers as well as over the whole process of pharmaceutical research, production, circulation, and utilization. Additionally, drug manufacturers are encouraged to form companies based on such ties as property rights, products, and marketing networks. Large drug wholesalers are encouraged to go to other regions to acquire municipal-level or county-level wholesalers and to convert them into regional distribution centers. Franchising of retail drugstores and counters for nonprescription drugs in franchise shops and supermarkets should also be promoted.

According to an interview with government officials in Shenzhen, the retail prices of drugs are national. Currently, medicine prices are administered by a three-tiered system: the State Planning Commission, the provincial price bureau, and the municipal price bureau. For major medicines, the State Planning Commission sets the highest retail price, and local authorities uniformly seek bids. For some drugs, the provincial price bureau sets the highest retail price.[77] Nonetheless, the study by the Social Security Research Institute also reveals that only a limited number of retail pharmacies have been certified as designated pharmacies. For instance, by the end of 2001, Shanghai had only about twenty drug retailers put on the list. In Zhenjiang, the certification of designated drug retailers had been delayed for four to five years, for it started to choose three drug retailers as test sites only in 2000.[78] In these two cities, the health-insurance department is under the Ministry of Health, and the certification of designated health entities is clearly affected by the interest of the department, which has manifested in the serious delay of the certification of designated drug retailers and enterprise-run clinics.[79] Actually, relatively strict restrictions have been imposed on the prescriptions filled by designated drug retailers. For example, in Changshu, every prescription may not cost more than 30 yuan, and only 250 cheap, effective, and relatively safe medicines are available. On the contrary, pharmacies at hospitals may sell 1,500 designated drugs.[80]

To understand the progress of the reform of medicine production and circulation system, the following report should be informative. In September 2003, the Shanghai government implemented six measures to support the development of economical drugstores (经济药房) and, thus, to reduce the prices of medicines. When economical drugstores appeared in Shanghai, the prices of medicines sold in 300 of its 1,500 drugstores plummeted. One of the measures was the inclusion of economical drugstores into the list of designated drugstores. To be certified as a designated drug retailer, the economical drugstore must have a business area of at least 1,000 square meters; four professional pharmacists (职业药师), six pharmacists (药师), and ten trainees (药士); and inexpensive medicines. It was expected that the certification of economical drugstores would affect hospital dispensaries, which sold 75 percent of the medicines, and in the case of designated drugs, almost enjoyed a monopoly. A survey based on a random sample of designated drug retailers had been conducted in Beijing, Shanghai, and Guangzhou. According to the survey, the amount of prescriptions filled at the designated drug retailers in Shanghai was noticeably smaller than those in Beijing and Guangzhou. On average, the designated drug retailers in Shanghai filled thirty-eight prescriptions per month, with a sales volume of less than 2,000 yuan, which amounted to only 0.8 percent of their total turnover. In addition, the number of designated drugs that these retailers carried was only 320, but the corresponding figures for Beijing and Guangzhou were 610 and 600, respectively.[81]

According to this report, there are several reasons for the unexpected outcome in Shanghai. First, hospitals used electronic or paperless prescriptions, and drugstores could not sell drugs to patients without prescriptions. Second, since profits from the selling of drugs were one of the main sources of income for hospitals, doctors would explain to their patients that although reimbursement could be obtained for drugs in the designated list, drugs outside the list were more effective, and the patients took their advice. Third, consumers had not yet grasped the idea of filling prescriptions at drugstores, and only 4 percent of the consumers in Beijing, Shanghai, and Guangzhou considered going to the designated drugstores when they purchased drugs. Fourth, the kinds of medicines on the designated list were few, as, for example, one drugstore carried more than 10,000 kinds of drugs, sold 4,000 to 5,000 kinds each day, but sold only 300 kinds of drugs listed in the catalog. Fifth, some patients explained that since it was difficult to buy all the required drugs at one drugstore, they filled the prescriptions at hospitals out of convenience. Sixth, most of the insurance subscribers were young or middle-aged people, and their physical conditions seldom made their annual expenses on medicines reach the standards of reimbursement, so they generally did not go to designated drugstores. As a result, many designated drugstores in Shanghai decided to return their business to that of general drugstores.[82] In other words, the provision of medical services has not yet separated from the selling of drugs.

The Reform of Rural Health Care

Along with the decollectivization of the rural economy and the reform of the urban health care system, the cooperative health care system supported by communes and production teams needs to be revised. In 2003, the Ministry of Health, Ministry of Finance, and Ministry of Agriculture jointly promulgated the Circular concerning the Establishment of a New-Style Rural Cooperative Health Care System.[83] According to this circular, the new-style cooperative health care system (新型农村合作医疗制度) is to be organized, guided, and supported by the government; funded from various channels (including the government and groups); and enrolled in voluntarily by individuals. That is, farming households may voluntarily participate in the new-style cooperative health care system by paying insurance premiums (农民以家庭为单位与个人缴费), township and village collectives must provide financial support (集体扶持), and the central and local treasuries must make allocations every year (政府资助).

Under this pooling scheme for mutual assistance, each individual is to pay at least 10 yuan as an insurance premium every year, but localities with better economic conditions may raise the amount of premium. As for workers employed by township and village enterprises, the county government will decide whether they should participate in the new-style cooperative health care system. Moreover, the collective economic entities in villages should provide appropriate financial support, while the county government should determine the amount of contribution. Furthermore, the local treasury should allocate, on average, at least 10 yuan for each enrollee every year, while the central government should allocate, on average, 10 yuan for each enrollee in the Western and Middle regions (excluding enrollees in the city).

The rural cooperative health care fund is used primarily for large medical expenses and hospitalization charges. Areas having the necessary conditions may set up a scheme combining large medical subsidies with small ones. In a given year, if an enrollee has not used any money from the fund, a regular physical checkup should be arranged for him or her. On one hand, the government of a province, autonomous region, or municipality directly under the central government should compile a catalog of basic medicines for reimbursement. On the other hand, the county government should determine the scope of payment, the payment standards, the amount of payment, and the examination items for the regular checkup.

Starting in 2003, each province, autonomous region, and municipality directly under the central government must select at least two to three counties (cities) (县市) as test sites and, having gained the necessary experiences, gradually expand the reform to other counties. Counties that do not have the necessary conditions may coordinate villages (townships) (乡〔镇〕) to implement the new system at the initial stage. The ultimate goal is to have the new system implemented nationwide by 2010.

Health Care Reform and Legislation

Like many other countries, China achieves policy objectives through the enactment and implementation of legislation. Moreover, over the years, China has adopted an incremental approach to effect reforms in various respects, such as economic reforms and labor reforms. With regard to health care, China has enacted various decrees and rules to implement the national policies of setting up the Basic Health Insurance system, reforming medical establishments, and improving the medicine production and circulation system. In 1994, the State Commission for Structural Reforms, Ministry of Finance, Ministry of Labor, and Ministry of Health jointly promulgated the Opinion concerning Test Sites for the Reform of the Health Care System for Staff and Workers, and the State Council allowed Zhenjiang and Jiujiang to become the pilot reform sites. After the experiences of Zhenjiang and Jiujiang proved successful, the State Council decided to expand the test sites by approving the Opinion concerning the Expansion of Test Sites for the Reform of the Health Care System for Staff and Workers in 1996. Two years later, having summed up the experiences of various test sites, the State Council promulgated the 1998 Decree in order to implement a uniform health insurance scheme nationwide. Based on the landmark 1998 Decree, the relevant ministries under the State Council, especially the Ministry of Labor and Social Security, have issued a number of accompanying rules to facilitate the implementation of the Basic Health Insurance.

Furthermore, although the State Council is the executive branch, it is also empowered to enact administrative regulations or issue decrees regarding matters falling within its administrative power. According to China's Constitution,[84] public health is a matter falling within the State Council's administrative power. Thus, the governing legislation on the health insurance reform has been the 1998 Decree. Nevertheless, since China has a large population with diverse cultures and disparate economic developments between regions, the State Council, at the central level, provides only general guidelines by promulgating administrative regulations and decrees, while local governments and local offices of the relevant ministries are empowered to implement national policies by enacting local statutes in light of local circumstances. The legislative approach taken by local authorities also mirrors the incremental approach of the central government. That is why some provinces or municipalities have passed provisional statutes prior to the promulgation of more lasting ones. These local statutory provisions not only set forth the necessary details for implementation but also provide for penalties in cases of noncompliance. Consequently, the discussion of health insurance reform in chapter 3, which focuses on the structures of local health insurance schemes, draws mostly on local statutes.

Notes

1. The Labor Insurance Regulations of the People's Republic of China, promulgated by the Government Administration Council on 26 February 1951 and amended on 2 January 1953.

2. The Circular on Several Questions regarding the Improvement of the Labor Insurance Health System for Staff and Workers, promulgated by the Ministry of Labor and the All China Federation of Trade Unions on 15 April 1966.

3. Xiao-wu Song and Hao Liu, "The Reform of the Health Insurance System and Accompanying Measures," in *Report on the Reform and Developments of China's Social Security System,* ed. Xiao-wu Song (Beijing: The Renmin University of China Chubanshe, 2001), 83–106, 85 (in Chinese).

4. *Ibid.*

5. *Ibid.*

6. *Ibid.*

7. The Directive regarding the Implementation of Publicly Funded Health Care and Prevention for State Personnel of the People's Governments, Parties, Organizations, and Institutions at Various Levels, promulgated by the Government Administration Council on 27 June 1952; the Measures for the Implementation of Publicly Funded Medicine and Prevention for State Personnel, promulgated by the Ministry of Health on 30 August 1952.

8. Song and Liu, (2001), 86.

9. Wei Yu, "The Important Issue of Enterprise Reform: Health Care Insurance System," in *The Reformability of China's State Sector*, ed. Guan-zhong J. Wen and Dian-qing Xu (Singapore: World Scientific Publishing Co., 1997), 433–63, 436.

10. *Ibid.*, 439.

11. Zi-you Yu, et al., "Health Care Expenses and Reform in China," *WCCS Papers* 7, no. 2 (March 1997), 1–14, 5.

12. *Ibid.*, 6–7.

13. *Ibid.*, 7.

14. *Ibid.*

15. Song and Liu, (2001), 87.

16. *Ibid.*, 88.

17. Dong-jin Wang, ed., *The Reform and Development of China's Social Security System* (Beijing: Falu Chubanshe, 2001), 278–279 (in Chinese).

18. *Ibid.*, 278.

19. *Ibid.*

20. *Ibid.*, 279.

21. Pei-yun Peng, "Opening Speech at the National Conference on the Expansion of Trial Work for the Reform of Health Care System for Staff and Workers, 8 April 1996,"

in *The Reform of the Health Care System for Staff and Workers,* ed. Distribution and Social Security Department of the State Structural Reform Commission, et. al, (Beijing: Gaige Chubanshe, 1996), 3–21, 4 (in Chinese).

22. Dong-jin Wang, "The Importance and Urgency of Sufficiently Understanding the Reform of the Health Insurance System for Urban Staff and Workers," *China Labor* 158, (January 1999), 4–7, 4 (in Chinese).

23. Wang, (1999), 4.

24. Song and Liu, (2001), 87.

25. Wang, (1999), 4; Peng, (1996), 4.

26. Song and Liu, (2001), 87–88.

27. Wang, (1999), 4; Song and Liu, (2001), 87–88.

28. Wang, (1999), 4.

29. Wang, (1999), 4; Song and Liu, (2001), 87.

30. Song and Liu, (2001), 87.

31. Peng, (1996), 4.

32. Peng, (1996), 4–5; Wang, (1999), 4.

33. Peng, (1996), 5; Song and Liu, (2001), 88.

34. Wang, (1999), 4.

35. Peng, (1996), 4.

36. *Ibid.*

37. *Ibid.*

38. Wang, (1999), 4; Peng, (1996), 5.

39. Jia-gui Chen and Yan-zhong Wang, "The Report on China's Urban Health Care System," in *China Social Security System Development Report 1997–2001,* ed. Jia-gui Chen (Beijing: Shehui Kexue Wenxian Chubanshe, 2001), 76–113, 81–82 (in Chinese).

40. Song and Liu, (2001), 89; Chen and Wang, (2001), 82.

41. Chen and Wang, (2001), 82.

42. *Ibid.*

43. Song and Liu, (2001), 90.

44. Chen and Wang, (2001), 82.

45. Song and Liu, (2001), 91; Wang (1999), 6.

46. The Opinion concerning Test Sites for the Reform of the Health Care System for Staff and Workers, promulgated by the State Commission for Structural Reforms, Ministry of Finance, Ministry of Labor, and Ministry of Health on 14 April 1994.

47. Wang, (1999), 6–7.

48. The Opinion concerning the Expansion of Test Sites for the Reform of Health Care System for Staff and Workers, promulgated by the State Commission for Structural Reforms, Ministry of Finance, Ministry of Labor, and Ministry of Health on 22 April 1996.

49. Wang, (1999), 6; Chen and Wang, (2001), 83.

50. The Decision concerning the Establishment of a Basic Health Insurance System for Urban Staff and Workers, promulgated by the State Council on 14 December 1998.

51. Lan-qing Li, Speech at the National Conference on the Reforms of the Basic HealthInsurance System and the Health and Medicine System for Urban Staff and Workers, 24–26 July 2000.

52. The Provisional Measures on the Administration of Designated Health Care Providers under the Basic Health Insurance for Urban Staff and Workers, promulgated by the Ministry of Labor and Social Security, Ministry of Health, and Chinese Medicines Management Bureau on 11 May 1999.

53. The Provisional Measures on the Administration of Designated Drug Retailers under the Basic Health Insurance for Urban Staff and Workers, promulgated by the Ministry of Labor and Social Security and Medicines Supervision and Management Bureau on 26

April 1999.

54. *See* the Circular regarding the Printing and Distribution of the State Catalog of Medicines for the Basic Health Insurance, promulgated by the Ministry of Labor and Social Security on 25 May 2000.

55. The Opinion on the Administration of Diagnosis and Treatment Items under the Basic Health Insurance for Urban Staff and Workers, promulgated by the Ministry of Labor and Social Security, State Development and Planning Commission, Ministry of Finance, Ministry of Health, and Chinese Medicines Management Bureau on 30 June 1999.

56. Peng, (1996), 7.

57. *Ibid.*, 8.

58. Li's speech at the National Conference.

59. Peng, (1996), 6.

60. *Ibid.*, 7.

61. *Ibid.*, 9.

62. Ritu Wu, "Establishing and Perfecting a System of Multi-Layered Health Insurance," *China Labor* 163 (June 1999): 11–12, 11 (in Chinese).

63. *Ibid.*

64. *Ibid.*

65. *Ibid.*

66. National Bureau of Statistics of China, *China Statistical Yearbook 2003* (Beijing, China Statistics Press, 2003), 844.

67. The Guiding Opinion concerning the Reform of the Urban Health and Medicine System, issued by the State Council Office of Structural Reforms, State Planning Commission, State Economic and Trade Commission, Ministry of Finance, Ministry of Labor and Social Security, Ministry of Health, Medicines Supervision and Management Bureau, and Chinese Medicines Management Bureau on 16 February 2000.

68. Social Security Research Institute, "An Investigative and Analytical Report on the Reform of the Health Insurance Systems in Zhenjiang, Changshu, and Shanghai," (unpublished report, the Ministry of Labor and Social Security of the People's Republic of China, 11 November 2001), 11 (in Chinese).

69. Wei Ding, "Documentary Facts about Shanghai's Reform of the Health System," *Renmin Ribao*, 28 August 2000 (in Chinese).

70. *Ibid.* Apparently, Ruijin Hospital had a lot of outpatients. Luwanqu Center Hospital did not have very good facilities. Shizheng Hospital was a small hospital.

71. Social Security Research Institute, (2001), 14.

72. *Ibid.*

73. *Ibid.*, 14–15.

74. Shu-duo Liu, "How to Change in the Reform of Hospitals?" *China Economic Times*, 24 March 2004. http://news.sohu.com (in Chinese).

75. *Ibid.*

76. *Ibid.*

77. Shenzhen City Social Security Administration Bureau and Shenzhen City Health Bureau, an interview with authors, Shenzhen, China, 19 November 2003.

78. Social Security Research Institute, (2001), 13.

79. *Ibid.*, 45.

80. *Ibid.*, 28.

81. Fan Zhang, "Behind the Desolation of Designated Pharmacies under HealthInsurance," *China Economic Times*, 24 March 2004. http://news.sohu.com (in Chinese).

82. *Ibid.*

83. The Circular concerning the Establishment of a New-Style Rural Cooperative Health Care System, promulgated by the Ministry of Health, Ministry of Finance, and

Ministry of Agriculture on 10 January 2003.

84. The Constitution of the People's Republic of China, adopted at the 5th Session of the 5th National People's Congress on 4 December 1982 and amended in 1988, 1993, 1999, and 2004, respectively.

Chapter 3

Health Insurance Reform in China

Among the three components of health care reform in China, the Basic Health Insurance system is the most controversial one. According to the Decision concerning the Establishment of the Basic Health Insurance System for Urban Staff and Workers (the 1998 Decree),[1] the primary objective of the system is to provide basic health care to urban workers through a socially pooled fund (mutual assistance) and personal medical accounts (individual responsibility). To implement the general principles enunciated in the 1998 Decree, provincial, municipal, and autonomous-regional governments have adopted various models in light of local circumstances. Accordingly, this chapter first explains the general framework of the Basic Health Insurance system and then introduces the major models for its implementation.

The General Framework

According to the 1998 Decree, the Basic Health Insurance applies to all urban hiring units (用人单位) and their workers, including state-owned enterprises, collectively owned enterprises, foreign investment enterprises, private enterprises, government organs, institutions, social organizations, and private non-enterprise entities (民办非企业单位). With respect to township enterprises and their employees as well as the owners and employees of individual economic entities (个体经济组织), the government of a province, autonomous region, or municipality directly under the central government should decide on their coverage. The Basic Health Insurance is to be composed of a socially pooled fund and personal medical accounts (统账结合). To finance the socially pooled fund and personal medical accounts, both the hiring unit and the worker are required to pay insurance premiums. Generally, the hiring unit should contribute about 6 percent of its total wages each month, whereas the worker is to contribute about 2 percent of his or her monthly wages. Nevertheless, the contribution rate can be adjusted in accordance with economic development. The insurance premium paid by the worker and a portion of the premium paid by the hiring unit must be credited to the worker's personal medical account. The proportion of the premium paid by the hiring unit that should be allocated to the personal medical account is to be determined locally with reference to such factors as the scope of payment of the personal medical account and the age of the worker. The remainder of the premium paid by the hiring unit will be allocated to the socially pooled fund. Moreover, the social-security-administration organ is to manage the socially pooled fund and personal medical accounts.

The principal and interest earned in the personal medical account belong to the worker. In fact, the money in the personal medical account can be used for medical expenses, can be carried forward, and can be inherited, but it cannot be withdrawn as cash or for other uses. Any medical expenditure incurred by the worker must be paid first from his or her personal medical account. If the money in the personal medical account is fully depleted, the worker will pay with personal funds whenever the medical cost is below the threshold of the socially pooled fund. The threshold of the socially pooled fund, which is the minimum amount that activates payment out of the fund, is about 10 percent of the average annual local wages, and the ceiling, which is the maximum amount that can be paid out from the fund, is about four times the average annual local wages. Although the socially pooled fund will pay medical costs above the threshold and below the ceiling, the worker also has to pay a certain proportion. The threshold, ceiling, and worker's share are to be determined in accordance with the principle of balancing revenue and expenditure.

Apart from incumbent workers, retired workers may also participate in the Basic Health Insurance scheme; however, they are not required to pay insurance premiums. Likewise, *xiagang* (下岗) workers, namely, workers who have been laid off due to enterprise restructuring, may participate in the Basic Health Insurance, but their insurance premiums are to be paid by re-employment service centers, using 60 percent of the previous year's average local wages as the base for computation (缴费基数). On the other hand, the medical benefits of retired cadres and old Red Army remain the same. That is, their medical expenses will be paid from the original sources. If the original financer, such as an institution, experiences financial difficulties, the same-level government is to provide assistance. The same will apply to certain disabled military personnel, and the social-security-administration organ is to maintain a separate account for them.

Under the Basic Health Insurance system, workers go to designated health care providers (定点医疗机构) for diagnosis and treatment. Thereafter, they can fill prescriptions at the hospital's outpatient pharmacy or designated drug retailers (定点零售药店). All designated health care providers are certified by the social-security-administration organs and must sign contracts with the social-security-administration organs in order to provide medical services.

Depending on medical needs, insurance subscribers can change health care providers either upward or downward in terms of the level or type of medical services. For instance, the insured may want to transfer from a level-one (township, village, or street) hospital to a level-two (district) hospital, from a level-three (municipal) hospital to a level-two hospital, or from a special hospital to a general hospital. To maintain the current level of health care in some industries, enterprises are allowed, as a transitory measure, to establish supplemental health insurance schemes. If the funding for enterprise supplemental health insurance is within 4 percent of total wages, it can be drawn from the "staff and worker welfare account." If the money in the "staff and worker welfare account" is not enough, enterprises may, subject to the approval of government, treat it as part of the operating cost.

Since the mid-1990s, local governments have adopted various models to implement the principle of combining a socially pooled fund with personal medical accounts. The common models include the Three-Phase Passage Model (三段通道式), Combined Boards Model (板块结合式), Three-Fund Management Model (三金管理式), and Pooling Scheme for Serious Illnesses (大病统筹).[2] These models were developed by local governments prior to the promulgation of the 1998 Decree. Thus, at the beginning of the health insurance reform, the distinctive features of these models were followed closely by the respective localities that had adopted them. However, as the 1998 Decree finalizes the general framework and local practices also evolve over time, existing features have been deleted, new features have been added, and overlapping features among various places have surfaced. For instance, Shanghai used to adopt the Pooling Scheme for Serious Illnesses, but the introduction of personal medical accounts as well as the establishment of a local additional health insurance fund have made its practice resemble the Three-Phase Passage Model. Similarly, Yantai has been one of the main representatives of the Three-Fund Management Model, but the replacement of the enterprise adjustment fund with the enterprise supplemental health insurance and the establishment of a large-amount medical relief fund have made its practice deviate from such model. Thus, the revised practices of various localities cast doubt on the continuous appropriateness of classifying them into these models and maintaining such nomenclatures. In the following discussion, the implementation mechanisms of four cities at various administrative levels are presented under the respective models that they have adopted or initially adopted.

The Three-Phase Passage Model

The so-called Three-Phase Passage Model refers to the three phases through which the insured pays his or her medical bills. In the first phase, the insured draws money from his or her personal medical account to pay for medical expenses. The second phase is self-payment, or out-of-pocket deductible. That is, when the personal medical account is depleted and there is insufficient money to pay for medical cost, the insured is required to pay an amount up to a certain percentage of his or her annual wages. The third phase is co-payment (activation of the socially pooled fund). That is, if the annual medical cost exceeds the balance of the personal medical account and a certain percentage of the insured's annual wages, the excess is to be paid jointly by the socially pooled fund and the insured. In general, the proportion to be paid by the insurance subscriber decreases as the amount of excess increases. Zhenjiang and Jiujiang have adopted this model. For the purpose of illustration, the following depicts the model adopted by Zhenjiang.

In 1994, Zhenjiang decided to experiment with the Three-Phase Passage Model by promulgating the Provisional Measures of Zhenjiang City on Health Insurance for Staff and Workers.[3] These measures mandated that the hiring unit was to pay 10 percent of its annual total wages as insurance premium, while the worker was to contribute 1 percent of his or her annual wages. Any medical expenses incurred by the worker must be paid first from his or her personal medical account (Phase One). If the money in the personal medical account was not sufficient, the worker had to pay with his or her own funds (Phase Two). However, if the amount of self-payment was greater than 5 percent of the worker's annual wages, the excess would be paid jointly by the socially pooled fund and the worker (Phase Three). Specifically, if the excess was 5,000 yuan or less, the amount of self-payment would be 10 percent; if the excess was greater than 5,000 yuan but up to 10,000 yuan, the amount of self-payment would be 8 percent; and if the excess was greater than 10,000 yuan, the amount of self-payment would be 2 percent.

After six years of experimentation, Zhenjiang's experiences cumulated in the passage of the Provisional Measures of Zhenjiang City on Social Health Insurance in 2001.[4] According to this new set of measures, Zhenjiang is to establish a multilayered Basic Health Insurance system, including the Basic Health Insurance, the hospitalization insurance (住院医疗保险), and the pooling scheme for the medical expenses of special groups (特殊人群医疗费用统筹). In terms of coverage, the Basic Health Insurance initially applies to the workers and retirees of such hiring units as enterprises, government organs, institutions, social organizations, and private non-enterprise entities; individual economic entities and their employees; and the self-employed, in the city. Other types of urban employees and those working in township enterprises are supposed to join gradually. The hospitalization insurance, however, applies to other types of urban employees who have not participated in the Basic Health Insurance, children of staff and workers, students, farmers, and the employees of a small number of enterprises that are suffering from financial difficulties. Similarly, the pooling scheme for the medical expenses of special groups applies to retired cadres, old workers who had participated in revolutionary work, and certain disabled military personnel.

Under the Basic Health Insurance, both the hiring unit and the worker have to pay insurance premiums. For the hiring unit, the base for calculating insurance premium is the previous year's total wages of its entire workforce, while the base for the worker is his or her previous year's total wages. If the total wages of the entire workforce is lower than 60 percent of the previous year's local annual wages of workers at the post, the 60 percent should be used as the base. For workers employed by private enterprises, township enterprises, or individual economic entities; the self-employed; etc., the base should be the previous year's local annual wages of workers at the post. For *xiagang* workers of state-owned enterprises who are receiving [lowest] livelihood guarantee allowance (〔最低〕生活保障费), that is, state poverty relief for urban residents, the base should be 60 percent of the previous year's local annual wages of workers at the post. The hiring unit must pay 9 percent of the base; the worker, 2 percent of the base; the self-employed, 11 percent of the base; and the *xiagang* workers, 11 percent of the base. Even unemployed people may continue to participate in the Basic Health Insurance. If an unemployed person is receiving unemployment benefits, he or she should pay 11 percent of the 60 percent of the previous year's local annual wages of workers at the post. If an unemployed person no longer receives unemployment benefits, he or she should pay 11 percent of the previous year's local annual wages of workers at the post. Upon retirement, if the hiring unit and the worker have continuously paid insurance premiums for thirty years or more (male), or twenty-five years or more (female), the retiree is entitled to receive benefits under the Basic Health Insurance without the need to pay insurance premiums. If insurance premiums have not been paid for the required number of years, the hiring unit and the retiree must make up for the deficiency by a lump-sum payment.

Once the required insurance premiums have been paid, the following proportion should be allocated to the personal medical account every year: if the worker is thirty-four years old or younger, 3 percent of his or her previous year's total wages should be allocated; if the worker is thirty-five to forty-four years old, 4 percent; and if the worker is forty-five years old or older, 5 percent. The remainder is to be allocated to the socially pooled fund. In the case of a retiree, the proportion to be credited to the personal medical account should be 6 percent of his or her previous year's total pensions. The principal and interest in the personal medical account belong to the insured and should be used only for medical expenditure; however, the balance of the personal medical account may be inherited. If the insured is transferred out of Zhenjiang, the balance of the personal medical account will also be transferred. If it is not possible to do the transfer, the balance may be allocated to the personal medical account of the insured's relative or be used up for his or her own medical cost.

In the case of an incumbent worker, the threshold of the socially pooled fund is 10 percent of his or her previous year's total wages. In the case of a retiree, the threshold is 5 percent of his or her previous year's total pensions. Any medical expenses incurred by the insured for outpatient services must be paid first from his or her personal medical account (Phase One). If the personal medical account is depleted and the medical cost is below the threshold, the insured must pay with personal funds (Phase Two). For outpatient expenses above the threshold, the socially pooled fund and the insured will co-pay (Phase

Three), and the respective proportions depend on the ranking of the health care provider. If the health care provider is a level-three hospital, the socially pooled fund will pay 65 percent, but the insured will pay 35 percent. If the health care provider is a level-two hospital, the socially pooled fund will pay 70 percent, while the insured will pay 30 percent. If the health care provider is a level-one hospital, the socially pooled fund will pay 75 percent, whereas the insured will pay 25 percent. Even so, the maximum amount paid by the socially pooled fund each year is 30,000 yuan. Moreover, if the number of years of paying premiums is less than five, the ceiling will be reduced by 5,000 yuan for each year of deficiency. For the general subscriber, the maximum amount of self-payment per year is 3,500 yuan, excluding expenses on special examination and treatment, controlled drugs, and drugs and services outside the scope of the Basic Health Insurance; expenses above the ceiling of the socially pooled fund; and payment incurred as a result of fewer than five years of paying insurance premiums. The expenses above 3,500 yuan will be borne by the socially pooled fund. Furthermore, the socially pooled fund is also used to pay for certain expenses relating to contagious diseases, birth-control surgery and sequelae, cancer treatment, chronic kidney degeneration, etc.

Likewise, regarding expenses incurred as a result of hospitalization, the insured must first draw money from his or her personal medical account. If the personal medical account is depleted and the hospital charges are below the threshold, the insured must pay with personal funds. Regarding any amount above the threshold, the socially pooled fund and the insured will co-pay in the following manner: If the excess is 5,000 yuan or less, the socially pooled fund will pay 80 percent while the insured will pay 20 percent; if the excess is greater than 5,000 yuan but up to 10,000 yuan, the socially pooled fund will pay 90 percent while the worker will pay 10 percent; and if the excess is greater than 10,000 yuan but up to the ceiling, the socially pooled fund will pay 95 percent while the insured will pay 5 percent. In the case of a retiree, the proportions of self-payment are half of the aforementioned percentages. Even so, if the one-time payment for special examination or treatment, such as ECT and TCT, during an outpatient visit or hospitalization is 300 yuan or more, the socially pooled fund will cover 70 percent while the insured will pay 30 percent.

Apart from the preceding insurance schemes, the overall social health insurance system of Zhenjiang contains other types of health insurance, including the pooling scheme for large medical expenses due to serious illnesses (大病高额医疗费用统筹), pooling scheme for hospitalization of the children of staff and workers and students (职工子女及学生住院医疗费用统筹), supplemental health insurance for special illnesses (特殊医疗补充保险), supplemental health insurance for hospitalization (住院补助保险), medical subsidies for public servants (公务员医疗补助), supplemental health care for model workers, experts, and graduate students (补充医疗保险照顾), and social medical relief (社会医疗救助). Except for the pooling scheme for large medical expenses due to serious illnesses, pooling scheme for hospitalization of the children of staff and workers and students, and social medical relief, these supplemental insurance schemes are designed to raise the level of health care for those who used to enjoy a higher level of health care (public servants), have made or will make contributions to society (model workers, experts, and graduate students), or would like to obtain additional insurance coverage. Since the pooling scheme for large medical expenses due to serious illnesses and the pooling scheme for hospitalization of the children of staff and workers and students are considered part of the Basic Health Insurance and the social medical relief fund is established for the disadvantaged, the following is a succinct account of these three insurance schemes.

First, those who participate in the Basic Health Insurance must also enroll in the pooling scheme for large medical expenses due to serious illnesses. The worker must pay 5 yuan as monthly insurance premium, whereas the retiree must pay 4 yuan. If the insured's accumulated medical expenses exceed the ceiling of the Basic Health Insurance (30,000 yuan), this socially pooled fund will be used to cover 95 percent of the excess. If the insured has paid premiums for five years or more, the maximum amount of payment is 50,000 yuan. If the insured has paid premiums for less than five years, the maximum amount of payment will be reduced by 10,000 yuan for each year of deficiency.

Similarly, the pooling scheme for hospitalization of the children of staff and workers and students applies to preschool children and students from primary school to university. For students, the insurance premium is 34 yuan; for preschool children, the insurance premium is 46 yuan. The ceiling of this pooling fund is 100,000 yuan. If the hospital charges are 1,000 yuan or less, the fund will reimburse 65 percent; if the charges are from 1,001 to 5,000 yuan, 70 percent; if the charges are from 5,001 to 10,000 yuan, 80 percent; if the charges are from 10,001 to 30,000, 90 percent; and if the charges are from 30,001 to 100,000, 95 percent. If the amount of self-payment exceeds six months' worth of the previous year's average social wages, the excess will be paid from this socially pooled fund.

On the other hand, the social medical relief fund is financed by a yearly transfer of 2 percent of funds from the pooling scheme for large medical expenses due to serious illnesses, allocations from the Treasury, and donations. Workers and retirees who are being provided with the lowest livelihood guarantee for urban families are entitled to receive medical relief. More specifically, if they have already participated in the Basic Health Insurance and the amount of self-payment is more than 1,000 yuan but less than 3,500 yuan, the social medical relief fund will pay for such an amount. If they have not yet enrolled in the Basic Health Insurance, the social medical relief fund will pay the fees for their participation in the hospitalization insurance.

The social health insurance of Zhenjiang applies only to Chinese workers. For the time being, foreign workers and those from Hong Kong, Macau, and Taiwan are not covered. Moreover, insurance for maternity, work-related injury, or occupational disease is regulated separately. In 2002, Zhenjiang had 418,000 participants in the Basic Health Insurance, and the participatory rate of workers amounted to 95 percent. The premium-paying rate was more than 95 percent. The amount of self-payment constituted 16.3 percent of the total amount of medical expenditures.[5]

The Combined Boards Model

Literally, the word "boards" in the Combined Boards Model refers to boards or plates. These boards or plates, namely, health insurance schemes applicable to different types of participants, comprise the overall social health insurance scheme. Shenzhen and Hainan have adopted this model. For the purpose of illustration, the following explains the Combined Boards Model adopted by Shenzhen.

According to the Measures of the Shenzhen City on Social Health Insurance for Urban Staff and Workers,[6] the government is to establish such types of health insurance as the Basic Health Insurance, local supplemental health insurance (地方补充医疗保险), and maternity insurance. In addition, the government is to provide medical subsidies for public servants and encourage enterprises to establish supplemental health insurance. All types of hiring units—including government organs, institutions, social organizations, enterprises, private non-enterprise entities, and intermediaries (中介机构)—and their workers—including incumbent staff and workers, retired personnel, and people who have Shenzhen household registration and are receiving unemployment benefits—must participate in the Basic Health Insurance, local supplemental health insurance, and maternity insurance.

The Basic Health Insurance is composed of a socially pooled fund and personal medical accounts, whereas the local supplemental health insurance and maternity insurance consist only of socially pooled funds. The Basic Health Insurance has two forms—the comprehensive health insurance (综合医疗保险) and the hospitalization insurance (住院医疗保险). The comprehensive health insurance is designed for the following people: (1) incumbent workers who have Shenzhen or blue-stamp household registration; (2) retirees who had Shenzhen household registration prior to retirement and are receiving monthly old-age pensions from municipal social-security-administration organs (hereinafter s-retirees); (3) retirees who had Shenzhen household registration prior to retirement, have participated in old-age pensions organized by the industry, and are receiving monthly old-age pensions paid by the Guangdong Province Social-Security-Administration Organ (hereinafter i-retirees); and (4) other workers as prescribed by the government. Even so, workers who do not have Shenzhen household registration may also participate in the comprehensive health insurance if their hiring units apply.

On the other hand, the hospitalization insurance is designed for the following people: (1) workers who do not have Shenzhen household registration; (2) retirees who do not have Shenzhen household registration but are receiving monthly old-age pensions from the municipal social-security-administration organ; and (3) people who have Shenzhen household registration and are receiving unemployment benefits. Those who have enrolled in the comprehensive health insurance or hospitalization insurance should concurrently sign up for the local supplemental health insurance.

With respect to the comprehensive health insurance, the base for calculating the insurance premium follows: (1) if the insured is an incumbent worker, the monthly wages of the worker should be used as the base; (2) if the monthly wages of the worker are greater than 300 percent of the previous year's average monthly wages of urban workers in Shenzhen, the 300 percent should be used as the base; (3) if the monthly wages of the worker are lower than 60 percent of the previous year's average monthly wages of urban workers in Shenzhen, the 60 percent should be used as the base; (4) if the insured is an s-retiree, the monthly basic old-age pension should be used as the base; or (5) if the insured is an i-retiree, the previous year's average monthly wages of urban workers in Shenzhen prior to retirement should be used as the base. If the insured is an incumbent worker, the insurance premium is 8 percent of the base, of which the hiring unit shoulders 6 percent and the worker contributes 2 percent. For the insurance premium of an s-retiree, the social-security-administration organ is to pay 11.5 percent of the base and list the payment as expenditure from the basic old-age pension mutual fund. For the insurance premium of an i-retiree, the original hiring unit is to make a one-time payment prior to retirement in the amount of the base x 11.5 percent x 12 months x 18 years.

The entire amount of insurance premium paid by the insured worker is allocated to his or her personal medical account. As to the insurance premium paid by the hiring unit or the social-security-administration organ, 30 percent will be allocated to the worker's personal medical account if he or she is younger than thirty-five years old; 40 percent if he or she is thirty-five to forty-four years old; and 50 percent if he or she is forty-five and older. If the insured is an s-retiree, 60 percent of the insurance premium will be allocated to his or her personal medical account; if the insured is an i-retiree, the amount to be allocated to his or her personal medical account is equal to the previous year's average monthly wages of urban workers in Shenzhen x 11.5 percent x 60 percent. The remainder of the insurance premium paid by the hiring unit or social-security-administration organ goes to the socially pooled fund. The insurance premium paid by the hiring unit should be listed as cost; the government should list it as operating cost for administrative affairs (行政事业经费); the insured should pay it before taxes.

If the insured is an incumbent worker, 90 percent of hospitalization expenses will be paid from the socially pooled fund, whereas the insured will pay 10 percent. If the insured is a retiree, 95 percent of hospitalization cost will be covered by the socially pooled fund, while the insured will pay 5 percent. For outpatient visits under the Basic Health Insurance or outpatient visits with prescription, diagnosis, and treatment listed under local supplemental health insurance, the insured must first pay from his or her personal medical account. If the personal medical account is insufficient, and the deficient amount in a medical year exceeds 10 percent of the previous year's annual wages of urban workers in Shenzhen, the socially pooled fund will cover 70 percent of the excess, and the insured will need to pay 30 percent. Moreover, if the social-security-administration organ approves large-scale medical equipment for testing or treatment during the outpatient visit, 80 percent of the medical costs will be covered by the socially pooled fund, and the worker will need to pay 20 percent. Similarly, when the insured, owing to medical needs and with the approval of the social-security-administration organ, uses special medical material or one-time medical material worth 1,000 yuan or more for diagnosis and treatment, or receives organ implant or transfer, the socially pooled fund will pay 90 percent of the State general-scale price or 50 percent of imported general-scale price. Furthermore, if the self-payment portion of the insured is relatively large, thereby causing his or her standard of living to go below the municipal lowest level of livelihood guarantee, the insured may apply for subsidies from the social-security-administration organ.

The payment ceiling of the socially pooled fund is four times the previous year's average annual wages of urban workers in Shenzhen and must be in line with the length of enrollment. Specifically, if the insured has been continuously enrolled for less than half a year, the payment ceiling is 0.5 times the previous year's annual wages of urban workers in Shenzhen. If the length of enrollment is at least six months but less than one year, the payment ceiling is one time; if the length of enrollment is at least one year but less than two years, the payment ceiling is two times; if the length of enrollment is at least two years but less than three years, the payment ceiling is three times; and if the length of enrollment is three years or more, the payment ceiling is four times.

Regarding the hospitalization insurance, the base for calculating the insurance premium should be the previous year's average monthly wages of urban workers in Shenzhen. For a worker who does not have Shenzhen household registration, the hiring unit is to pay 0.8 percent of the base as insurance premium. For a retiree who does not have Shenzhen household registration but is receiving monthly old-age pension from the municipal social-security-administration organ, or for a person who has Shenzhen household registration and is receiving unemployment benefits, the municipal social-security-administration organ is to pay 0.8 percent of the base as insurance premium and list it as expenditure from the basic old-age pension mutual fund or the unemployment insurance fund. All of the insurance premiums are allocated to the socially pooled fund; there are no personal medical accounts. As to expenses incurred as a result of hospitalization, 90 percent will be paid from the socially pooled fund, while the worker is required to pay 10 percent. If a retiree has been hospitalized, 95 percent of the expenses will be paid from the socially pooled fund, while the retiree will pay 5 percent. Except for certain types of outpatient visits approved by the social-security-administration organ, the insured has to bear the medical cost for outpatient visits.

If the insured has Shenzhen household registration and has been continuously enrolled in the Basic Health Insurance for one year or more, and no hiring unit pays insurance premiums for him or her during a change of job, he or she may continuously pay insurance premiums for a maximum period of three months. Nonetheless, if the insured or hiring unit ceases paying insurance premiums, the insured will not be entitled to insurance benefits, except for the money in the personal medical account, starting from the first day of the following month. Furthermore, if the insured leaves Shenzhen, the balance of his or her personal medical account will be transferred to the social-security-administration organ where he or she has household registration. If the place where the insured has moved has no such organ, the balance will be distributed to the insured as a one-time payment. If the insured dies, the balance will be distributed to his or her heirs. If there are no heirs, the balance will be transferred to the socially pooled fund.

In the case of the local supplemental health insurance, the bases for calculating the insurance premium are the same as those of the Basic Health Insurance. If the insured is a subscriber of the comprehensive health insurance, the insurance premium will be 0.5 percent of the base. If the insured is a subscriber of the hospitalization insurance, the insurance premium will be 0.2 percent of the base. If the insured is an incumbent worker, the hiring unit will pay the insurance premium. For retirees and those who have Shenzhen household registration and are receiving unemployment benefits, the source and means for paying the insurance premium are the same as in the case of the comprehensive health insurance and hospitalization insurance. No personal medical accounts are to be established; all of the insurance premiums are allocated to the local supplemental health insurance fund. The local supplemental health insurance fund will bear 85 percent, while the insured will pay 15 percent, for the following: (1) medical cost under the Basic Health Insurance in excess of the payment ceiling of the socially pooled fund, and (2) hospitalization expenses for prescription, diagnosis, or treatment listed under the local supplemental health insurance. The payment ceiling of the local supplemental health insurance is in line with the length of enrollment in the Basic Health Insurance. Specifically, if the insured has been continuously enrolled in the Basic Health Insurance for at least half a year but less than one year, the payment ceiling is 50,000 yuan; if the length of enrollment is at least one year but less than two years, the payment ceiling is 100,000 yuan; if the length of enrollment is at least two years but less than three years, the payment ceiling is 150,000 yuan; and if the length of enrollment is three years or more, the payment ceiling is 200,000 yuan.

The maternity insurance covers medical cost for testing, delivery, post-delivery visit, and birth-control surgery. Workers who have Shenzhen household registration should also participate in the maternity insurance. Under the Basic Health Insurance, local supplemental health insurance, and maternity insurance, appointment fees; expenditures on cosmetics, preventive medicine, PET, glasses, and hearing-aid; medical expenses incurred as a result of traffic accident, suicide, and fighting; etc. are not covered. In addition, these insurance schemes are not applicable to foreign workers and workers from Hong Kong, Macau, and Taiwan. Even so, the health care of the employees of individual economic entities who have Shenzhen household registration should be handled with reference to these insurance schemes.

An interview conducted in 2003 with government officials from the Shenzhen City Social-Security-Administration Bureau and Shenzhen City Health Bureau[7] reveals the following findings: The Basic Health Insurance has been extended to private enterprises, but it does not cover the family of workers; however, there is a pooling scheme for family members of the employees of government organs and institutions. At the time of the interview, the number of insurance subscribers was about 1.6 million, covering all workers and retirees who had Shenzhen household registration. The premium-paying rate was 99 percent, the highest in the country. The expenses covered by the Basic Health Insurance include basic medicines, basic diagnosis and treatment, and basic medical equipment. Medical services and drugs beyond the coverage of the Basic Health Insurance are paid for by the insured or from the original financial sources. Compared with enterprise workers, public servants have lower wages. Thus, medical subsidies are provided to public servants in order to maintain their pre-reform level of health care. If the insured leaves Shenzhen, his or her personal medical account will also be transferred; if the insured moves to a rural area, he or she will receive cash instead. Nowadays, workers who do not have Shenzhen household registration may also participate in the comprehensive health insurance if their hiring units are willing to do so. If enterprises do not pay insurance premiums, they will be imposed a fine; if enterprises do not pay and their workers have incurred medical expenses, they will have to pay on behalf of the workers.

The Three-Fund Management Model

To implement the Basic Health Insurance system, Qingdao and Yantai of Shandong Province adopted the so-called Three-Fund Management Model in the mid-1990s. According to the Provisional Measures of the Qingdao City on Health Insurance for Enterprise Staff and Workers,[8] insurance premiums paid by the hiring unit and the workers were to be allocated to three accounts. The first account was the socially pooled fund (社会统筹金), which was to be managed by the health-insurance organ and used for serious illnesses. The second account was the personal medical fund (个人账戶金), which was to be managed by the hiring unit on behalf of the worker and used for common or minor illnesses. The third account was the hiring-unit adjustment fund (单位调剂金), which was to be managed by the hiring unit, supervised by the trade union or congress of staff and workers, and used primarily as subsidies. Hence, the hiring unit and health-insurance organ jointly managed the health insurance scheme.

Although the participatory rates of enterprises in Qingdao and Yantai reached 93 percent and 96 percent, respectively, and the premium-paying rate to the socially pooled fund was over 90 percent, enterprises facing financial difficulties had not made sufficient contributions to the hiring-unit adjustment fund and personal medical fund, thus making reimbursement for medical expenses in arrears.[9] Moreover, since enterprises were still involved in the administration of health insurance, the objective of removing the social security burden from enterprises was frustrated, and the problem of workers receiving unequal treatment among enterprises could not be resolved.[10] Consequently, the Three-Fund Management Model was adopted for the transition from traditional health care to the reformed health care system.[11]

Having obtained more experience in health insurance reform, Qingdao and Yantai have revised their health insurance schemes. Their current implementations of the Basic Health Insurance reflect the national policy of socializing the administration of health insurance. In particular, the hiring-unit (or enterprise) adjustment fund has been replaced by the hiring-unit (or enterprise) supplemental health insurance, which is a voluntary program to be adopted by the hiring unit. For illustration purposes, the following discussion will depict the model adopted by Yantai.

According to the Measures of the Yantai City on the Implementation of the Basic Health Insurance System for Urban Staff and Workers,[12] all types of hiring units, including state-owned enterprises; collectively owned enterprises; foreign investment enterprises; enterprises funded by overseas Chinese from Hong Kong, Macau, and Taiwan; private enterprises; government organs; institutions; social organizations; and private non-enterprise entities and their workers must participate in the Basic Health Insurance. Moreover, the Basic Health Insurance will be gradually extended to township enterprises, urban individual economic entities, and their workers. Furthermore, the Basic Health Insurance is also applicable to workers who have urban household registration but work in township enterprises as well as retired personnel.

The Basic Health Insurance is composed of a socially pooled fund and personal medical accounts. Both the hiring unit and the worker must pay insurance premiums. The hiring unit must contribute 8 percent (7 percent after two years) of its total wages, while the worker is to contribute 2 percent of his or her wages. The contribution rate, subject to government approval, may be adjusted in accordance with economic development and the revenue and expenditure of the insurance fund. Retired workers, however, do not need to pay insurance premiums. If the wages on which the insurance premium is to be calculated are lower than 60 percent of the previous year's average local wages, the base for calculating the insurance premium should be the 60 percent. Enterprises that have been certified by the labor and social-security-administration department as "enterprises facing financial hardships" may pay 5.2 percent of the total wages as insurance premiums, which will be allocated to the socially pooled fund; however, their workers do not need to pay insurance premiums.[13]

As regards the insurance premium paid by the hiring unit, 65 percent should be allocated to the socially pooled fund, and 35 percent to the personal medical account. Nonetheless, this ratio may be adjusted in accordance with the revenue and expenditure of the insurance fund. Based on the principles of efficiency and fairness, and taking into account care for retired personnel, the monthly amount that should be transferred to the personal medical account is to be computed in accordance with the following formulae:

Incumbent worker:
Age coefficient x (Age of the worker - 17) + Coefficient of wages on which insurance premium is based x Base on which monthly insurance premium is calculated+ Base on which monthly insurance premium is calculated x 2%

Retiree:
Age coefficient x (Age of the retiree -17) + Pension coefficient x Total amount of pension each month

On the other hand, the entire amount of the insurance premium paid by the worker is to be allocated to the personal medical account.

The personal medical account is to be used for outpatient visits as well as hospitalization expenditure that should be paid by the worker. The principal and interest in the personal medical account belong to the worker. The money in the personal medical account must be used for medical purposes, but the balance can be carried forward or inherited. If the worker changes job, he or she should go through the formalities of transferring the personal medical account. If the worker moves to another place, he or she may request a lump-sum payment or the transfer of his or her personal medical account.

The payment threshold of the socially pooled fund follows: 8 percent of the previous year's average local wages in the case of a level-one hospital; 10 percent in the case of a level-two hospital; and 12 percent in the case of a level-three hospital. The payment ceiling of the socially pooled fund is four times the previous year's average local wages. However, certain medical expenses will not be paid from the socially pooled fund, for example, those incurred as a result of traffic accident, medical incident, crime, brawl, and suicide. The socially pooled fund is to be used primarily for hospitalization and outpatient visits based on a designated list of illnesses. In one medical year, if the amount of hospitalization expenses above the threshold each time reaches 5,000 yuan, the socially pooled fund will pay 70 percent; more than 5,000 yuan but less than 10,000 yuan, the socially pooled fund will pay 75 percent; and more than 10,000 yuan and up to the ceiling, the socially pooled fund will pay 80 percent. In the case of retired workers, the aforementioned ratios will be increased by 10 percent. For outpatient visits based on a designated illness, the socially pooled fund will pay 75 percent; for retired personnel, 80 percent.

The newly insured, including those who have discontinued the insurance for one year or more but have later re-enrolled, are entitled to receive benefits from the socially pooled fund after they have paid insurance premiums for one year; if they have paid for less than one year, the socially pooled fund will pay only 50 percent.[14] Nonetheless, the Basic Health Insurance does not cover maternity and work-related injury. If the worker participates in social security schemes for maternity and work-related injury, the medical expenses will be paid from the socially pooled funds established for maternity and work-related injury. If the worker does not participate in those insurance schemes, the expenses will be paid from the original financial sources.

Furthermore, enterprises that have the necessary conditions are allowed to establish enterprise supplemental health insurance (企业补充医疗保险). The Guiding Opinion regarding the Establishment of Enterprise Supplemental Health Insurance[15] provides that if the funding is within 4 percent of the total wages, it may be listed as part of the cost, without the need to obtain government approval. In addition, the measures for the administration of the enterprise supplemental health insurance should be adopted by the congress of staff and workers, the trade union, or the meeting of shareholders or of the board of directors (in stock enterprises) and reported to the same-level offices of the Ministry of Labor and Social Security and Ministry of Finance. The funding in the enterprise supplemental health insurance should be used as: (1) subsidies when the worker or retiree faces a heavy financial burden after his or her money in the Basic Health Insurance Fund and large-amount medical relief fund (discussed next) has been used up in one medical year; (2) subsidies when scientific and technical talents, model workers, key managers, etc. have to make personal payments for medical caretakers; and (3) any other medical fees as determined by the congress of staff and workers, the trade union, or the meeting of shareholders or of the board of directors. The enterprise supplemental health insurance is to be managed by the enterprise or centrally managed by the industry concerned, or, upon entrustment, by the local health-insurance organ. The financial condition of the enterprise supplemental health insurance must be reported to the entire body of workers or the congress of staff and workers.

For expenses above the payment ceiling of the socially pooled fund, the large-amount medical relief fund (大额医疗救助金) should be established. The insured is to contribute 2.5 yuan per month, but the insurance premium is paid in a lump sum every March. This fund covers 90 percent of any amount above the ceiling, while the insured has to pay 10 percent. The maximum amount of payment per year is 150,000 yuan. Moreover, to raise the level of health care, the hiring unit and the worker may also subscribe to commercial health insurance.

By the third quarter of 2003, Yantai had 11,058 hiring units, 632,364 workers, and 135,022 retirees participating in the Basic Health Insurance.[16] From April 2003 to March 2004, the payment threshold of the socially pooled fund was 500 yuan for a level-one hospital, 600 yuan for a level-two hospital, and

700 yuan for a level-three hospital; designated hospitals that had not been appraised were treated as level-two hospitals; and the payment ceiling was 32,200 yuan.[17]

The Pooling Scheme for Serious Illnesses

Generally, the Pooling Scheme for Serious Illnesses refers to the establishment of a socially pooled fund that is used to pay for medical expenditure incurred as a result of serious illnesses. This model has such an appellation principally because no personal medical accounts are set up for the subscribers and social pooling is the dominant characteristic. From May 1996 to November 2000, Shanghai conducted health care reform in three phases. In 1996, Shanghai established the socially pooled fund for hospitalization due to serious illness.[18] The hiring unit contributed 4.5 percent of its total wages to this insurance fund, to which 1 percent of the basic old-age pension fund was also allocated.[19] The worker paid 8 percent, but the retiree paid only 4 percent.[20] The threshold for level-one hospitals was 1,500 yuan; 2,000 yuan for level-two hospitals; and 2,500 yuan for level-three hospitals.[21] Both the worker and the hiring unit had to pay medical expenses below the threshold. For any amount above the threshold, the socially pooled fund was to pay 85 percent. The remaining 15 percent was to be paid by the hiring unit and the worker (7.5 percent) or the retiree (3.75 percent).[22] Subsequently, in 1997, Shanghai established the socially pooled fund for outpatient and emergency services due to serious illnesses.[23] The hiring unit contributed 1 percent to the insurance fund, to which 1 percent of the basic old-age pension fund was also allocated.[24] Likewise, in 1998, Shanghai established the socially pooled fund for retirees who need outpatient and emergency services.[25] Under this insurance scheme, 50 percent of the medical cost of a retiree was socially insured.[26] In other words, during this period, Shanghai took a wait-and-see approach toward the establishment of personal medical accounts. As such, Shanghai was one of the main representatives of the Pooling Scheme for Serious Illnesses.

In October and November 2000, Shanghai finalized its implementation plans for the Basic Health Insurance by promulgating the Measures of the Shanghai City on the Basic Health Insurance for Urban Staff and Workers[27] and the Detailed Rules of the Implementation of the Measures of the Shanghai City on the Basic Health Insurance for Urban Staff and Workers.[28] These statutory provisions institutionalize personal medical accounts and the local additional health insurance fund (地方附加医疗保险), which have made Shanghai's implementation practice resemble the Three-Phase Passage Model. The following discussion, therefore, will highlight the major provisions of Shanghai's latest insurance scheme.

In Shanghai, the Basic Health Insurance is to be extended to the staff and workers of enterprises, government organs, institutions, social organizations, and private non-enterprise units, including the retirees. However, foreign workers and workers from Hong Kong, Macau, and Taiwan are excluded from coverage.

Financially, the Basic Health Insurance consists of a socially pooled fund and personal medical accounts. Both the worker and the hiring unit are required to pay insurance premiums. The base on which the insurance premium of the worker is to be calculated is the previous year's average monthly wages. If the previous year's average monthly wages of the worker is greater than 300 percent of the previous year's average monthly local wages, the excess will not be counted toward the base. Nonetheless, if the previous year's average monthly wages is less than 60 percent of the previous year's average monthly local wages, an amount equal to the 60 percent will become the base. The incumbent worker is to pay 2 percent of the base as an insurance premium, while the retiree does not need to make individual contributions. The base on which the hiring unit is to calculate its insurance premium is the sum of all the bases on which the insurance premiums of workers are to be computed. The hiring unit is to pay 10 percent of the base as insurance premium for the Basic Health Insurance and 2 percent as insurance premium for the local additional health insurance.

The insurance premium paid by the worker is to be credited to his or her personal medical account. The money in the personal medical account can be carried forward or inherited. A portion of the insurance premium paid by the hiring unit is to be allocated to the worker's personal medical account, while the remainder goes to the socially pooled fund. The amount to be allocated to the personal medical account depends on the worker's age and whether the worker is at the post or is retired. For a worker who is at the post, the percentage to be allocated to his or her personal medical account is 0.5 percent of the previous year's average annual local wages if the worker is thirty-four years old or younger; 1 percent if the worker is thirty-five to forty-four years old; and 1.5 percent if the worker is forty-five years old or older. In the case of a retiree, the hiring unit is to allocate to his or her personal medical account 4 percent of the previous year's average annual local wages if the retiree is seventy-four years old or younger, but 4.5 percent if the retiree is seventy-five years old or older.

Under this insurance scheme, the insured may go to designated health care providers for diagnosis and treatment. To fill prescriptions, the insured may go to the outpatient pharmacies of designated health care providers or designated drug retailers. In the case of incumbent workers, the expenses for outpatient and emergency services as well as prescriptions at designated drug retailers are to be paid from the personal medical account. Likewise, the expenses incurred by retirees for outpatient and emergency services as well as prescriptions at designated drug retailers are to be paid from the personal medical account. On the other hand, the socially pooled fund is to be used for paying hospital charges. In the case of incumbent workers, the payment threshold of the socially pooled fund is 10 percent of the previous year's average annual local wages. In a given year, if the worker is hospitalized for treatment or observation, the socially pooled fund will pay 85 percent of the amount above the threshold. The remainder and any amount below the threshold are to be paid from the accumulated balance of the personal medical account. If the money in the personal medical account is insufficient, the worker will have to pay on his or her own. Likewise, in the case of retirees, the threshold of the socially pooled fund is 5 percent of the previous year's average annual local wages if the worker retired prior to 31 December 2000; 8 percent if the worker joined the workforce before 31 December 2000 and retired after 1 January 2001; and 10 percent if the worker joined the workforce and retired after 1 January 2001. In a given year, if the retiree is hospitalized for treatment or observation, the socially pooled fund will pay 92 percent of the amount above the threshold. The remainder and any amount below the threshold are to be paid from the accumulated balance of the personal medical account. If the money in the personal medical account is insufficient, the retiree will have to pay on his or her own. The payment ceiling of the socially pooled fund is four times the previous year's average annual local wages.

The local additional health insurance fund is used to pay outpatient and emergency fees upon the depletion of the personal medical account and hospital charges above the ceiling of the socially pooled fund. As to hospital charges above the ceiling of the socially pooled fund, 80 percent will be paid from the local additional health insurance fund, and the insured will pay the remainder. If there is insufficient money in the personal medical account to pay for outpatient and emergency services, the shortage, except for expenses incurred at designated drug retailers, will be paid in the following manner, depending on whether the insured is an incumbent worker or a retiree, as well as the age of the insured (whether the insured is an old (two categories), middle (three categories), or new person). For workers who were born before 31 December 1955, and joined the workforce prior to 31 December 2000, the insured will pay an amount up to 10 percent of the previous year's average annual local wages, and for the remaining shortage, the local additional health insurance fund will pay 70 percent while the insured will pay the rest. For workers who were born between 1 January 1956 and 31 December 1965, and joined the workforce prior to 31 December 2000, the insured will pay an amount up to 10 percent of the previous year's average annual local wages, and for the remaining shortage, the local additional health insurance fund will pay 60 percent while the insured will pay the rest. For workers who were born after 1 January 1966, and joined the workforce prior to 31 December 2000, the insured will pay an amount up to 10 percent of the previous year's average annual local wages, and for the remaining shortage, the local additional health insurance fund will pay 50 percent while the insured will pay the rest. For workers who joined the workforce after 1 January 2001, the insured has to pay for the entire shortage.

In the case of retirees, if there is insufficient money in the personal medical account, the shortage will, except for expenses incurred at designated drug retailers, be paid in the following manner: For those who retired before 31 December 2000, the insured will pay an amount up to 2 percent of the previous year's average annual local wages, and for the remaining shortage, 90 percent will be paid by the local additional health insurance fund if the health care provider is a level-one hospital (85 percent if the health care provider is a level-two hospital, and 80 percent if the health care provider is a level-three hospital), and the remainder will be borne by the insured. For those who were born before 31 December 1955, joined the workforce before 31 December 2000, and retired after 1 January 2001, the insured will pay an amount up to 5 percent of the previous year's average annual local wages, and for the remaining shortage, 85 percent will be paid by the local additional health insurance fund if the health care provider is a level-one hospital (80 percent if the health care provider is a level-two hospital, and 75 percent if the health care provider is a level-three hospital), and the remainder will be borne by the insured. For those who were born between 1 January 1956 and 31 December 1965, joined the workforce prior to 31 December 2000, and retired after 1 January 2001, the insured will pay an amount up to 5 percent of the previous year's average annual local wages, and for the remaining shortage, 70 percent will be paid by the local additional health insurance fund if the health care provider is a level-one hospital (65 percent if the health care provider is a level-two hospital, and 60 percent if the health care provider is a level-three hospital), and the remainder will be borne by the insured. For those who were born after 1 January 1966, joined the workforce before 31 December 2000, and retired after 1 January 2001, the insured will pay an amount up to 5 percent of the previous year's average annual local wages, and for the remaining shortage, 55 percent of the amount will be paid by the local additional health insurance fund if the health care provider is a level-one hospital (50 percent if the health care provider is a level-two hospital, and 45 percent if the health care provider is a level-three hospital), and the remainder will be borne by the insured. For those who joined the workforce as well as retired after 1 January 2001, the insured will pay an amount up to 10 percent of the previous year's average annual local wages, and for the remaining shortage, 55 percent will be paid by the local additional health insurance fund if the health care provider is a level-one hospital (50 percent if the health care provider is a level-two hospital, and 45 percent if the health care provider is a level-three hospital), and the remainder will be borne by the insured.

Despite the preceding rules, if the outpatient expenses are for treatment of serious illnesses, that is, dialysis, chemotherapy, and radiotherapy, the socially pooled fund will pay 85 percent if the insured is an incumbent worker, but 92 percent if the insured is a retiree. The remainder will be paid from the accumulated balance of the personal medical account. If the money in the personal medical account is not sufficient, the insured will have to pay for the deficiency. Similarly, if the insured remains sick at home, 80 percent of the home-care (家庭病床) expenses will be paid by the socially pooled fund, while the remainder will be paid from the accumulated balance of the personal medical account. If the money in the personal account is still not sufficient, the insured will have to pay for the deficiency. Furthermore, the socially pooled fund will pay all the expenses for outpatient and emergency services as well as for hospitalization relating to type-A contagious diseases and birth-control surgery. However, the socially pooled fund will pay only 50 percent of any amount above the threshold for hospitalization due to work-related injury or occupational sickness. The remainder as well as the fees for outpatient and emergency visits will be paid by the hiring unit in accordance with state and Shanghai regulations.

The socially pooled fund, local additional health insurance fund, and personal medical account will not pay medical expenses incurred as a result of suicide, drug addiction, medical incident, traffic accident, etc. If the hiring unit and/or the insured do not pay insurance premiums or have not paid insurance premiums in full, the insured will cease to enjoy insurance benefits the next month. If the outstanding premiums are subsequently paid, the insured will resume enjoying benefits the following month. During the period of suspension of insurance benefits, the hiring unit has to pay medical expenses. If the hiring unit and the worker have paid insurance premiums for a total of more than fifteen years, the worker will be entitled to receive insurance benefits after retirement.

By the end of 2002, Shanghai had about 6.95 million subscribers to the Basic Health Insurance.[29] Apart from home care, Shanghai has also included elderly care (老年护理) to the coverage of its health insurance scheme.[30] Moreover, the mutual-assistance supplemental health insurance schemes organized by trade unions have also alleviated the financial burden of those who have serious illnesses.[31]

A Synopsis of Implementation Models

To implement the national policy of adopting the Basic Health Insurance system, some local authorities have concentrated on establishing the Basic Health Insurance while others have taken a broader perspective, that is, the establishment of a comprehensive social health insurance scheme. In terms of an implementation model, the Pooling Scheme for Serious Illnesses does not have the personal medical account, but other models have such a device. The absence of personal medical accounts reduces the overall administrative cost of the Basic Health Insurance. Moreover, under the Three-Phase Passage Model, outpatient expenses above the threshold are covered by the socially pooled fund, whereas under the Combined Boards Model, outpatient fees, after the depletion of the personal medical account, are to be paid by the insured unless, as in the case of Shenzhen, the amount of excess in a medical year exceeds 10 percent of the previous year's annual wages of urban workers. Thus, to an extent, the Three-Phase Passage Model provides better coverage. Regardless of what model is adopted to deal with the means of payment for medical expenditure, similarities and differences exist in the realization of the national vision. Indeed, although the particulars of various schemes are different, the overall frameworks of these four cities are similar. For instance, owing to disparate stages of economic development and diverse social conditions, different local schemes mandate different contribution rates, different percentages of payment from the socially pooled fund, different types of treatment for incumbent workers and retirees, and different packages of supplemental health insurance. Even so, commonalities can be found among various local insurance schemes.

First, self-payment and co-payment have been introduced to ease the financial burdens on the government and the enterprise. In respect of coverage, incumbent workers, retirees, and recipients of unemployment benefits are the major subscribers, while extension of coverage to the private and individual sectors is on the horizon. Since the insured is entitled to use a designated list of medical services or to fill prescriptions under a designated list of medicines, preventive medicine is not emphasized, and expensive medical services or medicines are beyond the scope of coverage, the objective of the reform is to provide only the basic level of health care. To promote the spreading of risks among members of the relevant community, socially pooled funds are established for various purposes, such as the pooling scheme for large medical expenses due to serious illnesses and the pooling scheme for the hospitalization of the children of staff and workers and students. In other words, the personal medical account is used for outpatient services and minor illnesses, the socially pooled fund under the Basic Health Insurance is used for hospitalization and serious illnesses, and other socially pooled funds are used for large outpatient fees and hospital expenses above the ceiling of the socially pooled fund. For the poor and needy, medical relief funds supported by the government and/or donations have either been established or put on the agenda. Furthermore, the personal medical account is treated as an asset of the insured. That is, the more the insured contributes, the more funds will be available for use or to be passed down to the next generation. In this connection, the concept of vesting has been introduced because a worker will be able to continue receiving insurance benefits after retirement only if he or she has paid insurance premiums for the required number of years.

Notwithstanding the sundry implementation schemes used by local authorities during the transition period, there appears to be a trend of convergence, that is, the local schemes are moving closer, in terms of both theory and practice, to the system envisioned by the State Council. In particular, the responsibility of administering health care is transferred from the hiring unit to a social agency (the socialization of the administration of health care). The Basic Health Insurance is designed to meet the basic medical needs of a large segment of society (the objective of "low-level and broad coverage"). To cater to the different medical needs of workers and retirees, local or enterprise supplemental health insurance, commercial insurance, mutual-assistance insurance organized by the trade union, medical subsidies for public servants, etc. are established or encouraged (the realization of a multilayered and pluralistic insurance system). Moreover, the portability of the Basic Health Insurance and the entitlement to continuous subscription during the period of job change promote labor mobility (the development of a labor market).

Successes and Challenges

After several years of health insurance reform, stories of success have spread across the country, even though problems and challenges have also unfolded. With respect to successes, since the Basic Health Insurance is meant to provide health insurance to a large segment of society—that is, broad coverage—municipalities have the mandate to extend insurance coverage to all urban workers and retirees in their respective localities. Some cities have succeeded in providing broad coverage, for example, the participatory rates of Zhenjiang and Shanghai in June 2001 were 90 percent and 97.2 percent, respectively.[32] Moreover, the introduction of the co-payment has reduced the financial burden of employers. For example, in the first half of 2001, Zhenjiang incurred more than 103 million yuan of medical expenses, of which 17.66 percent were paid by the subscriber, 0.27 percent were paid by the hiring unit, and 82.07 percent were paid by various health insurance funds.[33]

Furthermore, rising medical costs have been somewhat controlled because the requirement of self-payment not only has made insurance subscribers become more conscious of medical expenditure (on the demand side) but has also forced doctors to consider fee guidelines regarding prescriptions as the distribution of health insurance funds is linked up with their performance (on the supply side).[34] In this regard, Zhenjiang is also a good example because its medical costs increased at an average of 33.4 percent for the three years prior to the introduction of the health insurance reform, but the corresponding figure was reduced to an average of 12 percent for the five years after the reform.[35] At the same time, the health insurance reform has enhanced the ability of all workers to stand against risks, especially for workers employed by small- and medium-sized enterprises, primary and secondary school teachers, retirees, and patients suffering from serious illnesses.[36]

Since the administration of health insurance has been socialized and the procedure of reimbursement of medical cost has been simplified, enterprises have reduced the cost of administering health insurance and the concomitant conflicts between workers and enterprise-run clinics.[37] Indeed, the elimination of concerns about the loss of health care and old-age pensions, which used to be tied to employers, has also facilitated enterprise reform.[38] Moreover, with the socialization of the administration of health insurance funds, designated hospitals must acquire computer equipment and train the necessary personnel.[39] Shanghai, for example, has invested 60 million yuan in building an information management system. A portion of the funds was used to purchase computers for designated hospitals.[40]

Furthermore, the health insurance reform has fostered various kinds of competition among medical establishments, such as competition among hospitals inside the city and competition among hospitals in neighboring cities.[41] Competition, in turn, has raised the management level of the hospital leadership, strengthened the doctors' consciousness regarding medical expenses, and caused hospitals to improve their quality of services, including catering to the needs of patients, improving the environment of hospital wards, and buying new medical equipment.[42] In a survey conducted by the Social Security Research Institute under the Ministry of Labor and Social Security, about one-third of the respondents claimed that the quality of medical services had improved and the incidents of unwarranted prescriptions had decreased.[43]

Despite the preceding stories of success, the health insurance reform has also generated problems and challenges. These problems and challenges either are the legacies of the traditional health care system or result from the structural defects of implementation models or of the overall framework. In the first place, the health insurance reform is meant to control the increasing cost of health care. Toward this end, the reform has been focused on the demand side, namely, reducing spending on health care. To a certain extent, this objective has been achieved; however, the overall effect has not been great or as expected. First, the cost of medicines is still high because (1) hospitals depend on sale commissions to secure money for expansion, and (2) some manufacturers of medicines provide high sale commissions in order to obtain market share.[44] Second, since hospital charges commonly are not itemized,[45] the fees for medical services are nontransparent, which may result in overcharging. Third, the supervision and control over the behavior of health care providers has been ineffective. For example, in Shanghai, payment is made upon the provision of medical service; however, this clearing system, or accounting method, is ineffective in controlling the behavior of health care providers as well as the overall medical cost.[46] In fact, hospitals that have violated regulations are required only to refund the illegally obtained income without the imposition of a fine.[47] Fourth, subscribers have only limited information about medical establishments and their services, so they often choose health care providers on a trial-and-error basis, which increases transaction costs. Given that the increasing cost of health care is due primarily to the loss of control of health care providers, namely, the oversupply of medical services, control of the demand side only is not sufficient. Until now, the health care reform has been focused on exploring the concrete measures to implement the principle of combining a socially pooled fund with personal medical accounts.[48] To control both the supply and demand sides, however, the reform of health insurance must proceed concurrently with the reform of medical establishments.[49]

Under the Three-Phase Passage Model, the false use of health insurance cards by family members, colleagues, and people who are not yet retired is common.[50] This phenomenon results from the fact that some cards have no attached photos, and medical personnel are under no pressure to verify the identity.[51] Since "multiple persons use one account" (一账多用), some subscribers use up the funds in their personal medical accounts quickly.[52] Because the socially pooled fund is used to pay for any amount of self-payment above the threshold and below the ceiling, the cost of social security will increase and the transfer of outpatient costs among subscribers will happen.[53] The end result is the overspending of the socially pooled fund and the overdrawing of personal medical accounts, which affects the balance of revenue and expenditure of the overall health insurance fund.[54] For example, from 1995 to 1997, the balance of personal medical accounts in Zhenjiang was 62,250,000 yuan, but the socially pooled fund had overspent 57,880,000 yuan, which, in effect, had almost emptied the funds in the personal medical accounts.[55] This phenomenon occurred partly because enterprises facing financial difficulties had not paid insurance premiums in full and partly because the Three-Phase Passage Model has an inherent structural problem.[56]

On the other hand, under the Combined Boards Model, expenses for an outpatient visit or a minor illness are to be paid from the personal medical account and/ or by the worker. This tighter control on the demand side has not resulted in the overspending of the socially pooled fund and the overdrawing of personal medical accounts.[57] Nevertheless, since expenses for outpatient visits and minor illnesses are paid from personal medical accounts and the boundary between serious illness and minor illness is unclear, subscribers who should receive outpatient services often opt for hospitalization.[58] In a survey conducted by the Social Security Research Institute under the Ministry of Labor and Social Security, about two-thirds of the respondents agreed that since the balances in the personal medical accounts belonged to the subscribers and can be inherited, those with minor illnesses might not consult doctors.[59]

Apart from the Three-Phase Passage Model, another reason for the false use of health insurance cards is the existence of differential treatment under the current framework. Nowadays, different health care treatment exists between incumbent workers and retirees, between workers and their families, and between urban workers and workers who have no local household registration or are from the rural area. Since the 1998 Decree provides that retirees are not required to pay insurance premiums, the local implementation of the Basic Health Insurance, especially in the case of Shanghai, is tilted toward the retirees.[60] In Shanghai, subscribers receive different health care treatment, depending on the subscriber's age. However, retirees do not necessarily earn less than workers at the post, and the medical expenses for older people may not necessarily be higher than those of middle-aged or young people.[61] Thus, it has been argued that retirees should also pay insurance premiums.[62] Likewise, the Basic Health Insurance currently excludes family members of the worker from coverage. As such, the question is how the immediate family of a worker can obtain some kind of health insurance. In this regard, Zhenjiang's solution is to set up a socially pooled fund for children of workers and students. Furthermore, to reduce financial burden, local insurance schemes have not required enterprises to obtain health insurance for workers from the countryside. Similarly, if a subscriber ceases to pay the monthly premium, he or she will not be entitled to any benefits the following month. Hence, the Basic Health Insurance also put workers from the countryside as well as workers with low income in a disadvantageous position.

Last, the progress of the health insurance reform is unbalanced. Some cities have overinsured because too many insurance schemes are available, while others are still struggling with the establishment of a socially pooled fund and personal medical accounts. In this regard, Shanghai is a good example of overinsurance because its Basic Health Insurance, local additional health insurance, and supplemental insurance organized by the trade union together reduce the amount of self-payment to as low as 6 percent.[63] Apparently, Shanghai's inclusion of home care and elderly care into the coverage of health insurance does not take the increased burden of the socially pooled fund into consideration.[64] In the same vein, since the government runs mandatory supplemental health insurance schemes, there is not much room for the development of enterprise supplemental health insurance and commercial insurance.[65] Nonetheless, higher insurance premiums can affect the competitiveness of enterprises, and mandatory supplemental health insurance schemes interfere with the self-autonomy of enterprises.[66] Meanwhile, enterprise-run clinics are outside the list of designated health care providers, even though general practitioners or other medical personnel in enterprise-run clinics can provide initial consultation and the charges of enterprise-run clinics are more reasonable than hospitals.[67] Furthermore, there are no clear and systematic standards to determine what illnesses should be covered by the socially pooled fund. The inclusion of a certain illness may result from the vigorous lobbying of an interest group. For example, in Zhenjiang, the socially pooled fund covers kidney dialysis patients but not hepatitis patients.[68] Hence, a more balanced development of the Basic Health Insurance remains to be seen.

Notes

1. The Decision concerning the Establishment of the Basic Health Insurance System for Urban Staff and Workers, promulgated by the State Council on 14 December 1998.
2. Xiao-wu Song and Hao Liu, "The Reform of the Health Insurance System and Accompanying Measures," in *Report on the Reform and Development of China's Social Security System*, ed. Xiao-wu Song (Beijing: Renmin University of China Chubanshe, 2001), 83–106, 95 (in Chinese).
3. The Provisional Measures of the Zhenjiang City on Health Insurance for Staff and Workers, promulgated by the Zhenjiang City People's Government on 7 December 1994.
4. The Provisional Measures of the Zhenjiang City on Social Health Insurance, promulgated by the Zhenjiang City People's Government in December 2001.
5. Zhenjiang Medical Insurance Bureau, "A General Account of Health Care Reform," www.zjyb.gov.cn/ybjj.htm (accessed 24 August 2004).
6. The Measures of the Shenzhen City on Social Health Insurance for Urban Staff and Workers, promulgated by the Shenzhen City People's Government on 27 May 2003.
7. Shenzhen City Social Security Administration Bureau and Shenzhen City Health Bureau, an interview with authors, Shenzhen, China, 19 November 2003.
8. The Provisional Measures of the Qingdao City on Health Insurance for Enterprise Staff and Workers, promulgated by the Qingdao City People's Government on 3 August 1995.
9. Song and Liu, (2001), 97.
10. *Ibid.*, 98.
11. *Ibid.*

12. The Measures of Yantai City on the Implementation of the Basic Health Insurance System for Urban Staff and Workers, promulgated by the Yantai City People's Government on 21 September 2000.

13. "The Major Policies of the Yantai City on the Basic Health Insurance," http://ldyantai. gov.cn/content/oper_guide/index_medicalinsure_poliyc.jsp (accessed 24 August 2004).

14. *Ibid.*

15. The Guiding Opinion regarding the Establishment of Enterprise Supplemental Health Insurance, promulgated by the Yantai City People's Government on 8 July 2003.

16. "Statistical Data on the City's Health Insurance for the Third Quarter of 2003," http://ld.yantai.gov.cn/content/oper_guide/index_medicalinsure_poliyc.jsp?id=17930 (accessed 24 August 2004).

17. "The Major Policies of Yantai City on the Basic Health Insurance," http://ld.yantai. gov.cn/content/oper_guide/index_medicalinsure_poliyc.jsp (accessed 24 August 2004).

18. Lu-guo Dai, "The Guarantee of Medical Care Is Not a Dream," *China Labor* 182 (February 2001), 4–6, 4 (in Chinese).

19. *Ibid.*

20. *Ibid.*

21. *Ibid.*

22. *Ibid.*

23. *Ibid.*

24. *Ibid.*

25. *Ibid.*

26. *Ibid.*

27. The Measures of the Shanghai City on the Basic Health Insurance for Urban Staff and Workers, promulgated by the Shanghai City People's Government on 20 October 2000.

28. The Detailed Rules for the Implementation of the Measures of the Shanghai City on the Basic Health Insurance for Urban Staff and Workers, promulgated by the Shanghai City Health Insurance Bureau on 15 November 2000.

29. National Bureau of Statistics of China, *China Statistical Yearbook 2003* (Beijing, China Statistics Press, 2003), 849.

30. Social Security Research Institute, "An Investigative and Analytical Report on the Reform of the Health Insurance Systems in Zhenjiang, Changshu, and Shanghai," (unpublished report, the Ministry of Labor and Social Security of the People's Republic of China, 11 November, 2001), 28 (in Chinese).

31. *Ibid.*, 7.

32. *Ibid.*, 8.

33. *Ibid.*

34. *Ibid.*, 11.

35. *Ibid.*, 9.

36. *Ibid.*, 10.

37. *Ibid.*, 9.

38. *Ibid.*

39. *Ibid.*, 11.

40. *Ibid.*

41. *Ibid.*, 10–11.

42. *Ibid.*, 11.

43. *Ibid.*, 24–25.

44. Tong-xin Li, "What Are the Difficulties in Controlling Drug Prices?" *Shichangbao*, 29 June 2000 (in Chinese).

45. *Beijing Qingnianbao*, "The Latest Statistics of the Ministry of Health: The Average

Cost of a Doctor Visit Is 79 Yuan," 18 August 2000 (in Chinese).
46. Social Security Research Institute, (2001), 14.
47. *Ibid.*, 15.
48. Song and Liu, (2001), 101.
49. *Ibid.*
50. Social Security Research Institute, (2001), 27.
51. *Ibid.*
52. Song and Liu, (2001), 95.
53. Social Security Research Institute, (2001), 34.
54. Song and Liu, (2001), 94.
55. *Ibid.*
56. *Ibid.*
57. Song and Liu, (2001), 96.
58. *Ibid.*
59. Social Security Research Institute, (2001), 24.
60. *Ibid.*, 38.
61. *Ibid.*
62. *Ibid.*, 47.
63. *Ibid.*, 15.
64. *Ibid.*, 28.
65. *Ibid.*, 15.
66. *Ibid.*, 30.
67. *Ibid.*, 22, 44.
68. *Ibid.*, 19.

Chapter 4

Theoretical Approaches to Health Care Provision

Status of Theories

The social science literature of recent years demonstrates that there is widespread interest in social welfare provisions (their origins, contents, impacts, etc.) among scholars, with a variety of theoretical starting points. This is fuelled in part by the discovery that social needs (health, income security, etc.) have remained unmet in many parts of the world as many states feel forced to adopt policies of fiscal austerity. Governments and academics in developed nations have been debating the role of the state in the provision of social welfare, and whether the state will continue to play a prominent role in social welfare provision in the future. In the area of social security, in particular, scholars and policy makers across the globe are looking for innovative and effective ways to improve people's well-being. Essentially, they are posing the question of how to meet basic needs (health, nutrition, shelter, income, etc.) so that people are given reasonable protection from major life risks.[1] A diverse range of theoretical and ideological positions in social policy have been taken, yielding numerous insights and proposing a variety of answers to this question. There has thus been an "intensification of ideological competition between rival visions of the 'Good Society.'"[2] As health care is one of the mainstays of a nation's welfare system, it has become one of the core areas of study in social policy. In this chapter, we will review several key philosophical and theoretical orientations that govern the discussion of social welfare provisions. We will make use of these in discussing both the present development and the future direction of health care reform in China.

Four influential theoretical perspectives in social policy are examined in this chapter: state welfarism, the neo-liberalism, the welfare pluralism, and social developmentalism. In essence, these are normative theories that provide a value framework for social policy and help in identifying desirable policies.[3] They each present different views on the character, objectives, and directions of social welfare provisions. Each offers a prescriptive as well as a descriptive view of how social welfare provisions ought to be delivered and by whom.

It cannot be overemphasized that theories are integral to the study of social science. One can identify several types of theory in social policy analysis: descriptive, analytical, and normative. The goal of a descriptive theory is the explication of social events and processes, as they exist at one point or at specific points in time.[4] Descriptive theories of welfare purport to discuss and examine the key features and operations of a welfare system. Normative theories of welfare seek not only to explain but also to give directions or guidelines for actions that will lead to certain desired results. Normative theories aim to exert a more profound impact on the course of social policy development in particular countries.

In social policy analysis, normative and descriptive theories are often complexly intertwined and can be separated only for analytical purposes. That is to say, theories that purport to explain welfare evolution invariably contain a normative element or perspective: They are concerned with how the policy can be better shaped to address social issues, and vice versa. Regarding the importance of theories (descriptive or normative) in social policy, Robert Pinker[5] has this to say:

> We need, therefore, to construct different kinds of model and theory, which will complement those we already have by taking account of the diverse sentiments of ordinary people. This exercise is worth undertaking for its own sake in so far as it seeks to widen our knowledge of social reality as it is. It is also necessary if we wish to change that reality into something more akin to a particular normative model or ideal type.

There is a common theme running through these normative theories in social policy analysis: policy relevance. To be meaningful, these theories must address specific social needs with relevant policy prescriptions. As Mishra[6] argues, "the study of welfare is approached from an interventionist point of view: not academic knowledge per se but, rather, recommending a course of action or at least laying bare the choices facing a society." Thus, a strong element of pragmatism is embedded in both descriptive and normative theories in social policy.

Invariably, economic and social progress benefit from a plurality of theories, since such theories have exerted considerable influence over the development of social welfare in different countries at different times. In the following chapters, we will examine whether and how these theories have informed the development of health care in China in recent past decades.

State Welfarism

State welfarism analyzes the development of the welfare state with respect to the provision of public service goods. The underlying principle of state welfarism is that the state, and not the individual, should bear primary responsibility for personal well-being, and should therefore provide a variety of social services like health care to meet social needs. State welfarism sees health care and all other modes of social security as a necessity as well as a right.

State welfarism is intimately tied to the concept of welfare state. During the postwar period, the idea that government should undertake comprehensive social security programs was widely accepted, and throughout the world, particularly in industrialized countries, social security programs expanded rapidly. State intervention is generally seen as a corrective for market failings, but it is also an important means of engineering a more equal and fair society. Prior to the late 1980s, access to health care was, in the dominant ideological perspective of many countries, a right of citizenship.[7]

The term "welfare state" is much used to refer to those countries in which government intervenes intensively in the social policy arena. Johnson[8] observes that the term "welfare state" came into more general use as a convenient shorthand way of referring to the social and economic policy changes in Western communities. One frequently cited definition of the goals of the welfare state comes from Briggs[9]: A "welfare state" is a state in which organized power is deliberately used in an effort to modify the play of market forces in at least three directions: (1) by guaranteeing individuals and families a minimum income irrespective of the market value of their property; (2) by narrowing the extent of insecurity by enabling individuals and families to meet certain "social contingencies" (for example, sickness, old age, and unemployment), which lead otherwise to individual and family crises; and (3) by ensuring that all citizens without distinction of status or class are offered the best standards available in relation to a certain agreed range of social services.

In the British context, there were three objectives: to extend the range of social services, to maintain full employment, and to nationalize some industries. The welfare state in Britain has been identified with the implementation of the recommendations of Beveridge's celebrated *Report on Social Insurance and Allied Services*.[10] This report examined the deficiencies of existing services and outlined a plan to attack the "five giants": idleness, ignorance, disease, squalor, and want. The solution was based on a free national health service, free education, public housing, social insurance, social assistance, and government policies to maintain full employment. The result was to be a Britain without poverty or want. Other scholars such as Mishra[11] identified similar characteristics of the welfare state: a commitment to a national minimum standard of living, full-employment policies, universal social programs, progressive taxation, social protection as an entitlement, and the promotion of a national community and social solidarity.

Overall, the "Golden Age" of the welfare state brought about the following changes to advanced industrialized countries[12] (and these changes capture the essence of welfare states). First, rapid reforms led to the creation of a society based on the idea of shared citizenship of all its members. Second, there was a commitment to use resources toward rapid expansion in the breadth and coverage of social welfare. Third, there was a broad-based political consensus in favor of a mixed economy and a system of extended social welfare. Finally, there was a commitment to growth and full employment. Many countries in the developed world accepted this idea of an expanded role for the state in economic and social life.

Proponents of state welfarism support a comprehensive national health care model, or a system of insurance/social security (see table 4.1), that is based on the notion of rights of citizenship. They perceive health care as a national endeavor. This line of thinking is captured by the Canadian experience. Facing the pressures to reform its health care system in the twenty-first century, the Canadian government undertook a comprehensive study of its health provisions and came up with a detailed report on the future of health services. The government-commissioned Romanov Report[13], which investigated the future of health care in Canada, found that "the reality is that Canadians embrace medicare as a public good, a national symbol and a defining aspect of their citizenship." It contended that Canadians expect the medical system to guarantee them equal access to a common basket of medical care services of equal quality, regardless of where they live.

Advocates of this approach are unhappy with other solutions, such as market-based solutions or the pluralist route (to be discussed later). For instance, the Romanov Report[14] seriously questions other "radical" solutions for reforming health care put forward by conservative and international bodies (including ideas like user fees, medical savings accounts, de-listing services, increased privatization, and a parallel private system), because evidence has not been forthcoming to support these ideas. Romanov, a former premier of Saskatchewan (Canada), emphatically concludes that "There is no evidence these solutions will deliver better or cheaper care, or improve access (except, perhaps, for those who can afford to pay for care out of their own pockets)." On the other hand, researchers from this stand point to the positive impacts of universal health provisions in the welfare states. Studies (see, for instance, Lahelma et al.[15]) have found that the existing health care arrangements and institutions in the Nordic welfare states are proving effective in buffering against the structural processes, which have tended to widen health inequalities in the 1990s.

Neo-liberalism

The neo-liberal approach stands in opposition to the state welfarist view. It contends that there should be no more than a residual or minimal involvement of the state in the provision of welfare. Essentially, this perspective argues that the conditions of economic growth play the crucial part in shaping the roles of the state in society. Orthodox thinking in economic analysis explains that economic growth is

Table 4.1 A typology of social policy theories as applied to health care

Welfare system	Type 1 State Welfarism	Type 2 Neo-liberalism	Type 3 Welfare Pluralism	Type 4 Socialism	Type 5 Social Developmentalism
General definition of health	Health care as an insured/ guaranteed public good or service	Health care as an item of personal consumption	Health care as predominantly a consumer good or service	Health care as a state-provided public service	Health care as a public good that promotes people's well-being in conjunction with a dynamic process of economic development
Status of the physicians	State employees	Solo entrepreneur	Solo entrepreneur and/or member of various groups/ organizations	State employees	Various roles, serving as planner for social development
Role of medical professional associations	Moderate, subordinate to the state	Powerful groups	Influential	Weak or non-existent	Moderate
Ownership of health system	Mostly public	Private	Private and public	Entirely public	Public and private
Health financing	State expenditure	Individual responsibility	Both state and individual contributions	Entirely from the state	Diverse sources: state, community, individuals
Role of the polity/state in health care	Central	Minimal	As one of the actors in "welfare mix"	Total	Significant, aligning social and economic development
Countries	Canada, France, Japan, New Zealand, Spain, Yugoslavia	Chile	Switzerland, USA	USSR	East Asian nations (Singapore, etc.)

Adapted and revised from Mark G. Field's *Success and Crisis in National Health Systems*, 1989, p. 7.

achieved by private enterprise, the economic benefits of trade liberalization, and a restricted role for the state. The neoclassical economic perspective attributes the modern economic miracle to an unbridled capitalism free from the restrictive measures of state intervention and organized labor. It thus attaches great significance to the market and it is basically anti-statist.

Since the late 1970s, neo-liberalism has been in the ascendant, sharing a number of common tenets with orthodox development economics.[16] According to the proponents of neo-liberalism, economic growth should be given the highest priority on the assumption that high growth will automatically solve the social problems and result in widespread prosperity. Under the influence of neo-liberalism, countries are encouraged to exploit all their resources, and public goods are to be opened up to complete privatization. These policies are designed to provide a favorable climate for the private sector and to harmonize the business environment across countries.

At the core of the debate on state welfare analysis is the notion of privatization, the idea that the nongovernmental (private) sectors should take on more of what are currently governmental functions. With the rise of conservative governments in Britain and the United States in the 1980s, privatization has come primarily to mean two things: (1) any shift of activities or functions from the state to the private sector; and (2) more specifically, any shift in the production of goods and services from the public to the private sector.[17] Starr[18] distinguishes some normative theories justifying privatization as a direction for public policy. By far the most influential is the vision grounded in laissez-faire individualism and free-market economics that promises greater efficiency, smaller government, and more individual choice if only we expand the domain of property rights and market forces.[19]

In the British context, privatization of social services is viewed as a political strategy for diverting demands away from the state and thereby reducing government overload. This view is associated with recent neo-conservative thought. Keynesian economic policies and Beveridge-style welfare policies are held responsible in the postwar years for the growth of government. The massive expenditure of resources and effort is said to have brought a great deal of harm: Governments have become overloaded to the point of ineffectiveness. Furthermore, the growth of public expenditure has "crowded out" industrial investment in the market sector. The welfare state is not so much the victim of economic problems as their cause.

All in all, neo-liberal thinkers put forward a number of principles for social security provisions: Social security services like health care should be provided mainly by means of a competitive market; the state should withdraw entirely from social insurance; means tests should be in place to ensure that scarce public resources are targeted to those most in need of them; and the state should stick to the principle of "less eligibility" to avoid the problem of moral hazard.[20]

The neo-liberal perspective has now come to center stage in any discussion of health care reform.[21] The proponents of this approach lament the expansion of the welfare state after the Second World War, arguing that its development has become part of the problem rather than the solution. In the field of health, Spicker[22] argues that welfare states and their "healthfare programmes" have failed and have only exacerbated the problem of health care. Likewise, Colclough[23] argues for the privatization of health service provision.

For some time now, international organizations such as the World Trade Organization (WTO), the World Bank, and the International Monetary Fund (IMF) have been championing the cause of neo-liberalism in social policy. In recent years, the World Bank has increasingly been taking over the roles in health policy formerly played by the historically dominant World Health Organization (WHO), since the former is the leading financier of health-sector activities in developing countries.[24] For a long time, the policy of privatization has been a centerpiece of the World Bank's and the IMF's agenda. In the case of health care, they have pushed for a more market-oriented health care model to replace the public-financed health care system.[25] The rationale for this move is predicated on efficiency, increased competition, and the supremacy of the market as an allocation mechanism. In the 1980s, the World Bank[26] recommended several forms of privatization in the health sectors of developing countries: the introduction of "user fees" for health services, the promotion of health insurance schemes, and increased investment in private care.

There was a subtle change in the position of the World Bank in the 1990s, after it realized that the strategy of full privatization was not working in many parts of the world; recognizing the limitations of a purely economic approach to health care delivery, it took a less doctrinaire position on privatization. Nevertheless, the fact that many developed and developing countries (including Asian nations) have embarked on "market" reforms shows the influence of neo-liberal thinking. Reviewing the rise of the private sector in health care in Asia, Newbrander and Moser[27], attributed this expansion to the inability of governments to adequately finance health services, the poor performance of public health service delivery systems, and the desire to expand the choices available to patients.

Since the beginning of China's transition from a state-planned to a market economy, three important publications from the World Bank have endorsed a market-based approach in health care delivery: "*China: Long-term Issues and Options in the Health Transition,*" "*China: Issues and Options in Health Financing,*" and "*Financing Health Care: Issues and Options for China.*[28] It is worth noting that the report *Financing Health Care* is based on joint research collaboration between the World Bank and the Chinese government (Ministry of Health), along with numerous of independent health care experts and academics. As a result, the report is much more pragmatic than other publications by the World Bank. It addresses the key concerns in health care development in China. Not surprisingly, both its analyses and recommendations somewhat diverge from the traditional neo-liberal approach, probably due to a belief that reliance on for-profit private sector organizations would be a non-starter, given the current stage of China's economic and social development.

As noted previously, the World Bank earlier tried to popularize the idea of a market-based system in health services throughout the world. In the early 1990s, it published an influential work, "*Investing in Health,*" alerting governments across the world to the high costs of public-sector health care services. To counter public overload, supporters of the market-based approach claim that the most effective option is to define most health services as commodities and relegate them to the market sector.[29]The state's role should be confined to areas like immunization and sewage disposal.

Academics and think tanks committed to the ideology of neo-liberalism have also entered this debate and made a number of suggestions to the Chinese government. Michael Tanner[30], a director of health and welfare studies at the Cato Institute, based in the United States, argues that state provision of health care services inevitably leads to overconsumption, which in turn places upward pressure on health care costs. He contends that only market forces can provide for China's future health care and retirement needs. Moreover, a private system based on individual accounts and private investment can promote full participation by workers in China's economic system, accelerating the move to a "shareholder-based economy." Most important, it "can increase economic growth and assist economic restructuring."[31]

Welfare Pluralism

In recent decades, there has been substantial support for the perspective of welfare pluralism among social policy thinkers. In large part, the theory of welfare pluralism arises as a response to the crisis in the welfare state. To some welfare pluralists, the state in Western democracies that still delivers comprehensive welfare services is considered overbureaucratic, overcentralized, and overauthoritarian. Consequently, health and other social services and benefits are inadequate and of poor quality. This state system is seen to be unresponsive to people's varied and changing needs, and clients have little or no control over the services. Hadley and Hatch[32] criticized the centralized administrative systems in developed nations on four counts: noncompliance (problems of political and hierarchical control); inefficiency and ineffectiveness; bureaucratic ossification; and failure to gain public support and involvement.

Speaking of the rising popularity of the pluralist approach, Pinker[33] argued that the conditions seem to be ripe for the idea of pluralism because public confidence in both Marxism and classical political economy had been undermined. Many people believe that neither a planned nor a competitive economy works particularly well in regard to social welfare provision. Welfare pluralism acts as a form of "damage limitation" in which the deficiencies of one approach are more or less balanced by the strengths of others. The pluralist approach is attractive for another reason. Unlike the neo-liberal thinkers who advocate the privatization and commercialization of social services, theorists from the pluralist strand of thought have taken a more moderate position.[34]

Other academics, examining existing public sector provisions, "discover" that many publicly provided social welfare goods are in fact jointly provided and financed.[35] In the case of Britain, scholars such as Jane Lewis[36] have urged others to rethink the nature of the "welfare state." Lewis argues that the story of the modern welfare state should not be seen as a simple increase in state intervention. It is more accurate to see Britain as always having had a mixed economy, in which the voluntary sector, the family, and the market have played different roles in the provision of welfare over the years.

What unites these writers is the call for a pluralist form of welfare state, with the state playing a smaller role in the direct provision of social services but retaining its role in finance and regulation. As Johnson[37] succinctly puts it,

> The major debate is no longer about the relative merits of a market system as compared with a centrally planned system. The major questions now revolve around such issues as the most appropriate size and scope of the market, the degree of regulation that is thought to be desirable and the degree to which government ought to intervene to enhance certain groups' ability to participate in the market and modify market outcomes.

The theory of welfare pluralism does not offer a clear blueprint for welfare provision. Its philosophy is rather that each locality must work out for itself what particular balance of services most nearly meets its needs.[38] It is a prescription of the most general kind. Its message is that welfare services can be obtained from four different sectors—the government, the voluntary, the commercial, and the informal sectors.[39] In fact, this "new" theory of pluralism stresses the contributions of communities and the informal sector. As Cook and White[40] rightly argue, "what perhaps is new is the extent to which these activities [on the part of informal sector and community] are regarded as forming a legitimate component of a formal system of welfare provision which the state can complement, support, and promote, rather than being viewed as a separate, informal, and possibly inefficient system."

This perspective argues for a pluralistic health delivery model[41] on the premise that a public/private sector mix is the best way to deliver health care. In the context of developing countries, Mwabu, Hjerppe, Ugaz, and White argue for an integrative approach to social service provision on the basis that "the process of social provision is multidimensional, involving efforts of many providers—state, market, and civil society."[42] In the field of health care, this perspective argues for a pluralistic approach to provision.[43] Such a pluralistic approach is particularly likely to be effective if it is designed to benefit from the prudent application of the powers of the state, from the efficiency of the market, and from community initiatives.[44]

Proponents of the private sector provision of health services argue that welfare pluralism has the potential to facilitate the provision of high-quality curative services while allowing the public sector to divert its limited services to the poor and high-risk groups. However, the growth of the private-sector market in health is still a cause of concern for many analysts. On the downside, the rise of private delivery could create a two-tier health care system and the proliferation of health insurance schemes. Further, competition between the two sectors for health care personnel could easily lead to a rise in health care costs.[45]

In this perspective, a balanced and judicious public/private mix in health care provision represent the best option. There is no lack of supporters of a mixed model of welfare in East Asia. Looking at Asia as a whole, Newbrander and Moser[46] advocate the following measures to further the goals of pluralism: The public sector must increase its sources of financing; it must find ways to reduce the costs of health delivery systems through increased efficiency and effectiveness; and it must relinquish to the private health sector responsibility for the delivery of health services in certain segments of the market.

Has there been empirical evidence in support of welfare pluralism in China's health care delivery? In the literature on health care, supporters of welfare pluralism can point to studies that show the important role played by the informal sector and families. For instance, drawing on a 1992 survey of some 20,000 samples, Pei and Pillai[47] affirm the impact of family support (together with support from the state) on the well-being of the elderly in China. They find that factors such as pensions, health care, size of family, and living arrangements are found to be significantly related to the perception of happiness among aged people in China. Their findings indicate the resilience of family support (via health care) in the promotion of a sense of well-being among elderly Chinese.

Social Developmentalism

Social developmentalism is a more recent normative theory that has arisen in response to the neo-liberal critique of state welfare. Progressive policy analysts have been searching for a more appropriate and effective approach to social provision in the wake of the neo-liberal challenge to the welfare state. Academics such as Midgley[48] have called for the adoption of a developmental approach that will promote social development and be consonant with the need for continued economic development. Proponents of this approach believe that social developmentalism provides an appropriate normative basis for social welfare in all parts of the world.[49] They further point out that there have been enormous improvements in standards of living for many people around the world over the last fifty years due to an emphasis on social development. Importantly, social development offers strong grounds on which to challenge the neo-liberal claim that social expenditures harm the economy and that economic development requires retrenchment in social welfare.

The developmentalist approach originated in the developing nations in the middle decades of the twentieth century, when many newly independent states sought to adopt economic policies that would promote rapid industrialization, increased employment, and improvements in living standards but which would, at the same time, address pressing social problems.[50] As recently as 1995, the United Nations made a determined effort to reinvigorate these key ideals by convening the World Social Summit in Copenhagen.[51]

Social development emphasizes the social aspects of the development agenda by harmonizing social interventions and economic development efforts within a wider commitment to social change and progress. It calls on governments to emphasize social programs that are compatible with development. There are two underlying principles: first, economic development should be integrated and sustainable, bringing benefits to all citizens; and second, social welfare should be investment-oriented, seeking to enhance the capacity of all human agents to participate in the economy.[52] Midgley argues that "social development cannot take place without economic development, and economic development is meaningless if it fails to bring about significant improvements in the well-being of the population as a whole." [53]

The productivist welfare approach in social development emphasizes the adoption of social policies that strive to enhance human functioning and capabilities. Central programmatic provisions include investments in human capital, employment and self-employment programs, social capital formation, asset development, and the removal of barriers to economic participation.[54] Governments should direct the process of social development in ways that maximize the participation of communities, the markets, and individuals in the development process.

There are several programmatic features in this approach: the creation of social planning agencies, the improvement of people's lives through economic development, and a preference for social programs that contribute positively to economic development. The developmental approach emphasizes the following values: harmonization of economic and social goals, investment-oriented social welfare, people's participation, adequacy, equality, and promotion of social cohesion.[55]

A number of features are embedded in this approach. First, social development promotes a pluralistic and consensual approach to social welfare that transcends the historic welfare statism of the European nations, advocating the integrated involvement of state, market, and community. It proposes that governments direct the process of social development in ways that maximize the participation of communities, the markets, and individuals in both economic and social development. By involving many constituencies in both economic and social policy, the prospects of reviving solidarity and promoting social integration increase. In this approach, productivist social policies and programs transcend the remedial and maintenance-oriented preoccupations of conventional welfarist approaches and instead seek to invest in the capabilities of needy people to participate effectively in the productive economy.

Theorists from this stand point to the developmental experience of Asian states as illustrating the manner in which social investment serves to support the economy. Singapore, Taiwan, and South Korea are all authoritarian developmental states and pro-growth in orientation. Yet, these developmental states tend to have extensive social services in such areas as housing, education, and health. These social services are considered a social investment and a method of furthering their national economic development goals. The approach appeals to the developmental states in East Asia since these states emphasize the productive function of social welfare in the course of their economic development.

Social developmentalism has taken a pragmatic, middle-of-the-road approach to social policy. It is an approach "promoting a particular form of action for incorporation more widely in social work." [56] It differs from the neo-liberal stance in that it regards state welfare as indispensable, but it recommends organizing state welfare in such way as to foster economic development. For the proponents of social developmentalism, all social needs must still be met, the state still has a vital role to play, and formal institutional structures are still necessary for social development. Where they differ from those on the left of the political spectrum is in advocating the harmonization of economic growth with social development, thus implicitly rejecting the theory of class struggle advocated by the Marxists.

Relevance of Theoretical Perspectives to China's Health Care Reform

Following this short review of the major theories in social policy as applied to health care, we can now assess whether they aid our understanding of health care delivery and the possible health care reform directions in present-day China. In the earlier chapters, we have seen that the Chinese government, after its rise to power in 1949, provided its urban employees (civil servants and industrial workers in state-owned enterprises) with publicly funded health care through two major health programs: the Government Insurance program and the Labor Insurance program. The rural areas relied on collective insurance schemes.[57] A socialist form of the health care system emerged in the early 1950s.

Essentially, the Government Insurance program paid for the health care services for all government employees, their dependants, veterans, educators, and college students. The Labor Insurance program covered the employees and retirees of the state-owned enterprises as well as their dependants. It is worth noting that some collectively owned enterprises provided their employees with full or partial health care coverage benefits following the Labor Insurance program. Health services, along with pensions, sickness benefits, housing, etc., were part of a comprehensive, employer-based social security system that was meant to achieve the socialist goal of replacing privilege and inequalities in the distribution of resources and opportunities with social and economic equality.[58] The state played a very significant role in health care delivery.

However, as China's economy took a market-oriented direction in the early 1980s, both the Government Insurance program and the Labor Insurance program were eroded and threatened by several fundamental problems for the insured: low coverage, poor risk pooling, and the lack of the incentives and accountability needed for economic efficiency and quality of care.[59]These program inadequacies, along with other economic and political forces, prompted health care reforms, marked by a shift from state provision to a more market-oriented system with policy tools like user fees, private provision, and insurance schemes. Drawing on our theoretical discussions, we could characterize the Chinese case a shift from a socialist to a market-oriented provision of health care. In the eyes of welfare pluralists, the shift in health care policies in China—involving all sectors, the state, families, and the non-profit and the for-profit sectors—actually proves their case.

Health care reform in China can also be seen from a comparative perspective. Much has been written about post-socialist as against capitalist health care systems.[60]In their comparative analysis of public social security across the world, Dixon and Hyde[61] identify some significant health care characteristics in post-socialist nations. They contend that an ideology of "authoritarian reluctant individualism" gradually emerged in post-socialist nations when they realized and accepted state economic failure and turned toward a limited form of market ("market pragmatism") in the delivery of social security. These post-socialist states, while being authoritarian, continue to uphold these principles: the right to social security for all, public social security provisions for the vulnerable, and increasing individual responsibility to meet social security needs.

Did the Chinese case fit into this form of "authoritarian reluctant individualism"? In the case of Communist China, one would guess that the reality is much more complex than the situation discussed by Dixon and Hyde. One wonders whether the ideology of "authoritarian reluctant collectivism" can capture the full reality of public social security, because a constellation of social, economic, and political forces and ideologies are at work. One also wonders whether the principles of the right to social security and public social security provisions for the vulnerable are upheld in the case of health care.

Setting aside the question of which direction China is heading in health care reform, it is important to assess how these theories or ideologies have impacted the course of social security reform in China.

Following the economic opening in the late 1970s, China has been exposed to various ideological and philosophical forces (which we discussed earlier) that impinge on the social security (pension and health) reform process. In practical terms, scholars[62] have identified several potent lines of thinking in social security reform: pluralist, socialist, neo-liberal, and developmental. Needless to say, the socialist position emphasizes state responsibility and redistributive fairness as the guiding principles for the reform. Since China is still a socialist state, this position is popular among some groups (the Ministry of Labor, trade unions, civil servants, etc.).[63]

Not surprisingly, some scholars also subscribe to this view, insisting that the Chinese government should play a very active role in financing public health services. In large part, such sentiment is backed by the past achievements of the Chinese government. As Yang and associates[64]point out, China has developed the world's largest network of health care services, and the health status of its people has risen dramatically during the past four decades. The reasons for these achievements include an ideology of equity for all citizens and the near universal availability of adequate food, education, housing, jobs, transport, accessible and affordable treatment, and preventive health services.

Some authors on the right of the political spectrum have suggested that China must drop all socialist tenets and pursue the neo-liberal route. They urge that it must develop market-based health care systems based on individual accounts and private investments for providing old age and health protection. This would be one form of market liberalism whereby individuals would be ultimately responsible for their health care and retirement needs. The state would eventually play only a residual role in social services. Such a private delivery system would, the argument runs, actually increase economic growth and assist economic restructuring.

In the context of social security reform, international bodies such as the World Bank (i.e., *China 2020 Series*) have worked out a number of guiding principles for China: (1) unifying the pension system, bringing together enterprises and workers currently covered under separate plans into a single system with common standards; (2) reducing the pension burden by gradually increasing the retirement age, lowering the wage replacement rate, and indexing pensions to prices rather than wages; (3) introducing funded individual accounts to end the problems associated with the current pay-as-you-go system; and (4) ensuring an adequate real rate of return on pension funds.[65]

Evidently, a pension plan informed by these principles would be funded by a combination of the state, enterprises, and individuals themselves. These principles would be easy to apply to other areas of social security like health care and housing. The World Bank's proposal emphasizes financial sustainability (i.e., the rate of return and the setting up of individual accounts) and system unification. Similar ideas would be extended to health care reform, with the setting up of individual health accounts, reductions in state spending on health care, and emphasis on fiscal sustainability.

There are both strengths and weaknesses in this position. One must acknowledge that Chinese financing reforms of public health services (fixed budgets and fee charges, etc.) have had some positive impacts: improving the financial accountability of public health institutions, increasing the incentives for the public health institutions to improve their productivity as well as reducing the government's financial burden.[66] However, opponents of market-oriented financing reforms of public health services argue that such a system would bring some undesirable consequences in the form of escalating costs and reduced access. For instance, an empirical study done by Gao and his associates[67] showed that access of the urban population in China, particularly the poor, to formal health services has worsened and has become more inequitable since the early 1990s due to this market-oriented financing policy.

In contrast to these standpoints, a third option is now being debated in relation to China: a developmental statist stance,[68] which stresses market efficiency but seeks pragmatically to design pension and health schemes consistent with rapid economic growth, whether by statist or market means. White calls this approach "developmental statism" [69]and notes that it is already winning strong support in China. Advocates of this approach come from the areas of China where local governments are strongly "committed to organizing growth within their own bailiwicks and judge policy alternatives by this single criterion." [70]Their position is generally in line with the central aim of welfare developmentalism: enhancing the capacities of needy people to participate in the productive economy, the health service being one of the key enablers to materializing this goal.

As these three approaches are being hotly debated by Chinese officials as well as scholars, it is important not to lose sight of the welfare pluralist route, because there are sources of health care (in the market, voluntary, and informal sectors) outside the state.[71]Further, as a normative theory welfare pluralism is appealing because it recommends reliance on a "welfare-mix," i.e., diverse sources for the delivery of health services.

These are some of the strands of thinking that capture the attention of people in general as well as of officials, and which are having a strong impact on the course of social security policies as they are developed in China. It is important to be aware, however, that in the case of a particular social program like health care, these represent only some of the many factors that come into play in China. Other crucial factors like financial constraints, path dependency, interest group dynamics, political considerations, and social stability are equally important. Twenty-first-century China faces the following challenges in health care reforms: cost escalation, reductions in state spending, and increased private contributions. The formidable task for the Chinese government is to meet these challenges while maintaining social stability and so ensuring that economic development will not be easily undermined.

Notes

1. James Midgley, Martin Tracy and Michelle Livermore, eds., *The Handbook of Social Policy* (Thousand Oaks, CA: Sage Publications, 2000).

2. Gosta Esping-Andersen, et al., *Why We Need A New Welfare State* (Thousand Oaks, CA: Sage Publication, 2002).

3. Anthony Hall and James Midgley, eds., *Social Policy for Development* (Thousand Oaks, CA: Sage Publications, 2004).

4. Michael Martin and Jane Sell, "The Role of the Experiment in the Social Sciences,"*The Sociological Quarterly* 20, no.4 (1979): 581–590.

5. Robert Pinker, *Social Theory and Social Policy* (London: Heinemann, 1979), 135–136.

6. Ramesh Mishra, *Society and Social Policy* (London: Macmillan, 1981), 4.

7. Mark G. Field, ed., *Success and Crisis in National Health Systems: A Comparative*

Approach (New York: Routledge, 1989).

8. Norman Johnson, *The Welfare State in Transition: The Theory and Practice of Welfare Pluralism* (Sussex: Wheatsheaf Books, 1987); Idem., *Reconstructing the Welfare State: A Decade of Change 1980–1990* (Sussex: Wheatsheaf Books, 1990); Idem., ed., *Private Markets in Health and Welfare* (Oxford: Berg Publications, 1995).

9. Asa Briggs, "The Welfare State in Historical Perspective," *Europene de Sociologie* 2, no. 2 (1961): 212–258.

10. William Beveridge, *Social Insurance and Allied Services* (London: HMSO, 1942).

11. Ramesh Mishra, *The Welfare State in Crisis* (Brighton: Wheatsheaf Books, 1984).

12. Christopher Pierson, *Beyond the Welfare State* (Cambridge: Polity, 1991); Amartya Sen, *Development as Freedom* (New York: Anchor Books, 1999).

13. R. J. Romanow, *Building on Values: The Future of Health Care in Canada 2002*, www.healthcarecommission.ca/default.asp?DN=cn=2,ou=Stories,ou=Suite247, o=HCC (accessed 17 January 2003).

14. *Ibid.*

15. Eero Lahelma, et al., "Analysing Changes of Health Inequalities in the Nordic Welfare States," *Social Science and Medicine* 55 (2002): 609–625.

16. Midgley, Tracy and Livermore (2000).

17. Paul Starr, "The Meaning of Privatization," in *Privatization and the Welfare State*, ed. S. Kamerman and A. Kahn (Princeton, NJ: Princeton University Press, 1989), 15–48; Idem., "The Limits of Privatization," in *Privatization and Deregulation in Global Perspective*, ed. D. J. Gayle and J. N. Goodrich (New York: Quorum Books, 1990), 109–125.

18. Starr, (1989).

19. Kwong-leung Tang, "The Case for the Privatization of Social Welfare: Three Decades of Public Opinion from Great Britain and the United States," *Scandinavian Journal of Social Welfare* no. 6 (1997): 34–43.

20. John Dixon and Mark Hyde, eds., *The Marketization of Social Security: International Perspectives* (Westport, CT: Quorum Books, 2001).

21. Andrew C. Twaddle, "Health System Reforms: Toward a Framework for International Comparisons," *Social Science and Medicine* 43, no. 5 (1996): 637–654; Susan Giaimo and Philip Manow, "Adapting the Welfare State," *Comparative Political Studies* 32, no. 8 (1999): 967–1000, 967.

22. S. F. Spicker, "Going Off the Dole: A Prudential and Ethical Critique of the 'Healthfare' State," in *Reforming Health Care: The Philosophy and Practice of International Health Reform*, ed. David Seedhouse (Chicester: John Wiley & Sons, 1995), 131–142.

23. Christopher Colclough, ed., *Marketizing Education and Health in Developing Countries* (Oxford: Clarendon, 1997).

24. Mrigesh Bhatia and Elias Mossialos, "Health Systems in Developing Countries," in*Social Policy for Development*, ed. A. Hall and J. Midgley (Thousand Oaks, CA: Sage Publications, 2004), 168–204.

25. Twaddle, (1996); Wynand P. M. M. van de Ven, "Market-oriented Health Care Reforms: Trends and Future Options," *Social Science and Medicine* 43, no.5 (1996): 655– 666.

26. World Bank, *Financing Health Services in Developing Countries: An Agenda for Reform* (Washington, DC: World Bank, 1987).

27. William Newbrander and Patricia Moser, "Private Health Sector Growth in Asia: An Introduction," in *Private Health Sector Growth in Asia*, ed. W. Newbrander (Chichester: John Wiley & Sons, 1997a), 1–10.

28. *See* various reports issued by the World Bank: World Bank, *China: Long-Term Issues and Options in the Health Transition* (Washington DC: World Bank, 1992); Idem.,

Investing in Health: World Development Report (New York: Oxford University Press, 1993); Idem., *China: Issues and Options in Health Financing* (Washington DC: World Bank, 1996); Idem., *Financing Health Care: Issues and Options for China,* China 2020 Series, (Washington DC: World Bank, 1997).

29. Craig R. Janes, "The Health Transition, Global Modernity and the Crisis of Traditional Medicine: The Tibetan Case," *Social Science and Medicine* 48 (1999): 1803–1820.

30. Michael Tanner, "Using Market Mechanisms to Provide Retirement Security and Health Care in China," in *China in the New Millennium: Market Reforms and Social Development*, ed. James A. Dorn (Washington D.C.: Cato Institute, 1998), 319–330. Also see De-zhi Yu, "Market-Based Reforms and Changes in China's Health Care System," in *Social Provisions in Low-Income Countries: New Patterns and Emerging Trends*, ed. G. Mwabu et al. (Oxford: Oxford University Press, 2001), 265–287.

31. *Ibid.* Tanner, (1998), 330.

32. Roger Hadley and Stephen Hatch, *Social Welfare and the Failure of the State* (London: Allen & Unwin, 1981).

33. Robert Pinker, "Making Sense of the Mixed Economy of Welfare," *Social Policy and Administration* 26, no.4 (1992): 273–284.

34. Johnson, (1995).

35. Sarah Cook and Gordon White, "Alternative Approaches to Welfare Policy Analysis: New Institutional Economics, Politics, and Political Economy," in *Social Provisions in Low-Income Countries: New Patterns and Emerging Trends*, ed. G. Mwabu et al. (Oxford: Oxford University Press, 2001), 26–52.

36. Jane Lewis, *The Voluntary Sector, the State and Social Work* (Aldershot: Edward Elgar, 1995).

37. Johnson, (1995), 13.

38. Johnson, (1990, 1995).

39. Neil Gilbert, *Capitalism and the Welfare State* (New Haven, CT: Yale University Press, 1984).

40. Cook and White, (2001), 32.

41. Field, (1989), 3.

42. Germano Mwabu, et al., "Introduction: Context and Scope," in *Social Provisions in Low-Income Countries: New Patterns and Emerging Trends*, ed. G. Mwabu et al. (Oxford: Oxford University Press, 2001), 3.

43. Field, (1989), 3.

44. Mwabu, et al., (2001), 5.

45. William Newbrander and Patricia Moser, "The Future of Health Sector Reform in Asia," in *Private Health Sector Growth in Asia*, ed. W. Newbrander (Chichester: John Wiley & Sons, 1997b), 221–229.

46. Newbrander and Moser, (1997b).

47. Xiao-mei Pei and Vijayan K. Pillai, "Old Age Support in China: The Role of the State and the Family," *International Journal of Aging and Human Development* 49, no. 3 (1999): 197–212.

48. *See* James Midgley, *Social Development: The Developmental Perspective in Social Welfare* (Thousand Oaks, CA: Sage Publications, 1995); Idem., *Social Welfare in Global Context* (Thousand Oaks, CA: Sage Publications, 1997); Idem., "Growth, Redistribution and Welfare: Towards Social Investment," *Social Service Review* 73, no. 1 (1999): 1–12; James Midgley, "Globalization, Capitalism and Social Welfare: A Social Development Perspective," *Canadian Social Work Review* 17 (2000): 13–28; and Idem., "Poverty and the Social Development Approach," in *Poverty Monitoring and Alleviation in East Asia*, ed. Kwong-leung Tang and Chack-kie Wong (New York: Nova Science Press, 2003), 155–178. Also see Michael Sherraden, *Assets and the Poor: A New American Welfare*

Policy (Armonk, NY: M.E. Sharpe, 1991).

49. James Midgley and Michael Sherraden, "The Social Development Perspective inSocial Policy," in *The Handbook of Social Policy*, ed. J. Midgley et al. (Thousand Oaks, CA: Sage Publications, 2000), 435–445; Kwong-leung Tang and Raymond Ngan, "China: Developmentalism and Social Security," *International Journal of Social Welfare* 10, no.4 (2001): 253–259; Kwong-leung Tang and James Midgley, "Social Policy after the East Asian Crisis: Forging a Normative Basis for Welfare," *Journal of Asian Comparative Development* 1, no. 2 (2002): 301–318.

50. Tang and Midgley, (2002).

51. Midgley, (2003).

52. Midgley, (1995, 1997, 1999, 2003).

53. Midgley, (1997), 181.

54. Tang and Midgley, (2002), and Midgley, (2003).

55. Tang and Ngan, (2001).

56. Malcolm Payne, *Modern Social Work Theory* (Chicago: Lyceum Books, 1997), 213.

57. Marie L. Lassey, William R. Lassey and Martin J. Jinks, *Health Care Systems Around the World: Characteristics, Issues and Reforms* (New Jersey: Prentice Hall, 1997).

58. Alan Walker, *Social Planning: A Strategy for Socialist Welfare* (Oxford: Basil Blackwell, 1984).

59. Tang and Ngan, (2001).

60. Walker, (1984), and Lassey, Lassey and Jinks, (1997). Also see Anthony Cheung and Xing-yuan Gu, "Health Finance," *in Social Policy Reform in Hong Kong and Shanghai: A Tale of Two Cities*, ed. Linda Wong, Lynn White, and Shi-xun Gui (Armonk, NY: M. E. Sharpe, 2004), 23–52; James A Dorn, ed., *China in the New Millennium* (Washington DC: Cato Institute, 1998); Jane Duckett, "Political Interests and the Implementation of China's Urban Health Insurance Reform," *Social Policy and Administration* 35, no. 3 (2001): 290–306.

61. Dixon and Hyde, (2001).

62. Charles C. Griffin, *Health Care in Asia: A Comparative Study of Cost and Financing* (Washington DC: World Bank, 1992); Gordon White, "Social Security Reforms in China: Toward an East Asian Model?" in *The East Asian Welfare Model*, ed. R. Goodman et al. (New York: Routledge, 1998), 175–198; Zu-liu Hu, "Social Protection and Enterprise Reform," in *Enterprise and Social Benefits from Communism*, ed. M. Rein, B. Friedman and A. Worgotter (Cambridge University Press: Cambridge, 1998), 284–304; Solomon R. Benatar, Abdallah Daar, and Peter Singer, "Global Health Ethics: The Rationale for Mutual Caring," *International Affair* 79, no. 1 (2003): 107–138; Gerald Bloom and Xing-yuan Gu, "Health Sector Reform: Lessons from China," *Social Science and Medicine* 45, no. 3 (2000): 351– 360.

63. White, (1998).

64. Pel-lin Yang, Vivian Lin, and James Lawson, "Health Policy Reform in the People's Republic of China," *International Journal of Health Services* 21, no. 3 (1991): 481–491. Also see Xing-zhu Liu and J. L. Wang, "An Introduction to China's Health Care System," *Journal of Public Health Policy* 2, no. 1 (1991): 104–116; Russell Smyth, "Labor-Market and Social-Welfare Reform in the State-Owned Sector in China," *Journal of Developing Areas* 33, no. 2 (1999): 223–244; Gordon G. Liu, et al., and Tadashi Yamada, "Equity in Health Care Access: Assessing the Urban Health Insurance Reform in China," *Social Science and Medicine* 55, no. 10 (2002): 1779–1794.

65. World Bank, (1997).

66. Xing-zhu Liu and Anne Mills, "Financing Reforms of Public Health Services in China: Lessons for Other Nations," *Social Science and Medicine* 54, no. 11 (2000): 1691–1698.

67. Jun Gao, et al., "Changing Access to Health Services in Urban China: Implications for Equity," *Health Policy and Planning* 16, no. 3 (2001): 302–312.

68. White, (1998); Tang and Ngan, (2001).

69. White, (1998), 186.

70. White, (1998), 184–185.

71. Martin Powell and Martin Hewitt, *Welfare State and Welfare Change* (Buckingham; Philadelphia: Open University Press, 2002).

Chapter 5

Health Care Reform and Stakeholders' Opinions in Wuhan

Introduction

This chapter looks at health care reform, its central focus being the use of basic health insurance in the perception of two principal stakeholders—patients in hospitals and employees of employment units who have joined Basic Health Insurance. The chapter examines whether and how far health care reform has the support of its principal stakeholders.

The overall objective of health care reform in China is to provide better-quality medical services at a relatively cheap cost to satisfy the basic medical needs of ordinary people. As discussed earlier, health care reform consists of three major components: the introduction of a medical insurance program covering the basic medical needs of urban workers, the reform of medical establishments, and the reform of the medicine production and circulation system. These components are to be seen in the larger context of the policy and ideological assumptions that underpin them; hence, it is possible for us to understand whether health care reform has advanced primarily by looking at the shifts in policy and ideology. Survey findings should be a good source of information on this, because they detect people's subjective attitudes and thus reflect their policy and ideological preferences. In the present context, the findings of our social surveys can provide answers to the following two questions in connection with our inquiry into health care reform in China: First, do they reflect public endorsement of the policy shift that has seen the market, rather than the state, as bearing responsibility for meeting health care needs? Second, is this policy shift also accompanied by a profound shift in the mix of ideologies underpinning health care reform?[1]

In other words, not only are the findings from our social surveys used to examine the problems arising by reference to the explicit policy intentions, they are also used to examine whether and how far health care reform initiatives have achieved the underlying shifts at policy and ideological levels. We focus on the shift of health care responsibility from the employment units, generally regarded as a part of the state apparatus in China's old command economy, to the employees themselves, and how far this shift reflects the changing mix of ideologies underpinning the reformed urban health care system in China.

The Two Social Surveys and their Context—Wuhan City

Two medium-scale social surveys were conducted in December 2003 in Wuhan city, one aimed at urban employees, the other at hospital patients. Each has a sample size of just over 300 respondents—305 for employees and 302 for patients. A brief introduction to Wuhan city is presented first, followed by a description of the sampling procedures.

Wuhan is situated in the middle of Hubei Province in central China. It is a large mid-China city with a population of 7.8 million people (see the Location of Wuhan in China map). It is one of China's traditional manufacturing bases. For example, in 2004, nine out of every 100 cars manufactured in China came from Wuhan's Citroen-Dongfeng, a company set up with a combination of French and Chinese capital. It is also one of the biggest iron and steel industry bases in China.[2] Nevertheless, in comparative terms, Wuhan is one of China's less developed cities. In 2003, it was ranked fourteenth among nineteen big cities with subprovincial status in terms of residents' disposable annual income—its residents had an average income of 8,525 yuan, which is very close to the national average of 8,472 yuan. In Shenzhen, ranked the number-one city, the corresponding figure was 23,906 yuan, thus a wide income gap is found between the front runner and Wuhan.[3] In a number of other key indicators in 2003, Wuhan also reflects the urban average in China. For instance, the unemployment rate in Wuhan was 4.66 percent, compared with the national average of 4.3 percent; the Engel ratio, which measures the share of spending on food to total household spending, was 40.6 percent in Wuhan, compared with the national urban average of 37.1 percent; the sex ratio was 51.6 percent male and 48.4 percent female in Wuhan, compared with the national urban average figures of 51.5 percent and 48.5 percent. However, in terms of economic growth rate, Wuhan achieved a rate of 12.1 percent in 2003, somewhat higher than the national average of 9.1 percent in the same year.[4] In sum, while Wuhan lags well behind the burgeoning coastal cities such as Shenzhen and Shanghai, its economic development is more representative of the nation as a whole.

It was in 2003 that China's average per capita GDP (at current prices, not in terms of purchasing power parity) reached the US$1,000 threshold, implying that the average Chinese citizen has a decent living standard above subsistence level.

Location of Wuhan in China

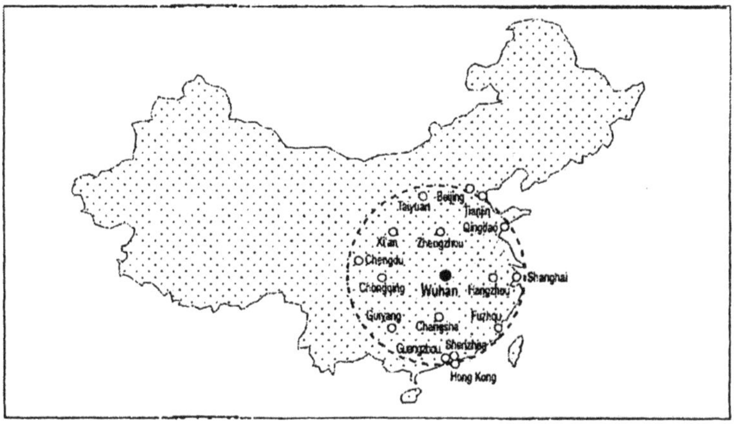

The residents of Wuhan were not exceptional in this respect. When our social surveys were conducted at the end of 2003, they enjoyed the lifestyle commonly enjoyed in cities in China at that time. For example, every 100 households in Wuhan possessed 38 computers, 115.4 air-conditioners, 136.2 color TVs, and 103 refrigerators.[5] The possession of these domestic appliances suggests that economic standards in Wuhan had been substantially improved over the reform era. Apparently, these are evidence of the trickle-down effect of the overall economic reform, which was first introduced experimentally in the southern Pearl River Delta, spearheaded by the setting up of "Special Economic Zones" like Shenzhen in the early 1980s, accelerated in the eastern coastal regions such as Shanghai in the 1990s, and spilling over into the less developed inner regions of mid- and western China throughout the process. Hence, although Wuhan has lagged behind the leading cities in economic development, its residents were nevertheless enjoying the fruits of economic reform at the time the surveys were conducted.

Not only has Wuhan lagged behind in terms of economic development, it is also one of the latecomers in health insurance reform, only introducing the Basic Health Insurance scheme at the end of 2001. In other words, it is a good case study to see how far health care reform has advanced in an economically less developed but strong manufacturing city in mid-China. Wuhan residents should have strong expectations of the state for health care protection, having previously enjoyed high levels of such protection under the command economy.

In 2003, when the two social surveys were conducted, Wuhan had an urban workforce of 4.12 million in a near eight-million strong population. According to government statistics, 1.31 million of its workers joined the new Basic Health

Insurance scheme; this means that by 2003, only one-third of Wuhan's urban workforce had basic insurance coverage. However, the annual rate of growth in coverage was enormous—an increase of 64 percent, or a half million in absolute numbers, over the previous year.[6] So, this mid-China big city was catching up fast. Indeed, it was only a few years before, in 1999, that Wuhan Municipal Government had set up the Medical Insurance System Reform Office (保险制度政革办公室) to coordinate all matters related to health care reform. On the basis of the findings of a comprehensive survey on the conditions of medical insurance in the city, a "Temporary Method" (暂行办法) for implementing health insurance was announced in the same year. Subsequently, a dozen preparatory documents complementing the implementation of medical insurance were circulated for comments before they became official in 2001 and 2002. They included the key document—*Basic Medical Health* (武汉市城镇职工基本医疗保险办法).[7] In the same year, the Wuhan Health Insurance Center (医疗保险中心), the administration organ of the city's Labor and Social Security Bureau (劳动和社会保障局), was established to implement all matters related to the city's Basic Health Insurance. Wuhan was hailed as one of the pioneers in the exploration of a number of new measures in health care reform—basic health insurance and health assistance schemes for government employees, the establishment of special clinics for chronically ill patients, the implementation of serious illness assistance, and the coordination of basic hospital care protection for employees in enterprises in difficulty.

In 2001, a new health insurance system was formulated in Wuhan. It comprises basic health insurance, serious illness insurance, supplemental medical insurance for enterprises, and serious illness assistance. Needless to say, the stakeholders of the two key schemes of the old health care system, Government Insurance, the publicly funded health system (see chapter 2), and Labor Insurance, have been encouraged to join the new system so that economies of scale can be achieved in the latter. In this regard, Wuhan has a multilayered new health insurance system and aims at dismantling the old one. The Wuhan Health Insurance Center is responsible for implementing health care reform in the city in line with the national plan for health care reform. In October 2001, the Municipal Government authorized the first batch of twenty-eight medical establishments, mainly hospitals, and twenty retail drugstores, to accept those insured for, respectively, medical treatment and the purchase of medicines.

Due to the fact that only a small proportion of the population in Wuhan had access to health care protection, a general household survey might not have been the best strategy to examine the effects of the new scheme. We therefore selected employees as the first group of respondents, because Basic Health Insurance is principally an employment-based program. The disadvantage of this choice is that it would leave out the unemployed and *xiagang* workers from the survey. On the other hand, if the major stakeholder group for medical insurance, the employees, are dissatisfied with the health care reforms, it can be assumed that the unemployed and laid-off workers are likely to be even more dissatisfied. In other words, the employee group can serve as a proxy for their worse-off fellow residents. The second group of respondents were the hospital patients; they were directly affected by the new reform measures. Both groups are principal stakeholders of the new reform measures. For instance, employees have to contribute from their income to secure insurance benefits, while patients are affected by reforms in hospitals and in the control of drug and price lists. There may be an overlap between the two respondent groups—for example, some employees may also come to the hospital for treatment. Nevertheless, as they were interviewed in different settings—employees in their workplaces and patients in hospitals—they are treated as distinct groups. They were interviewed using the same set of core questions, but the socio-demographic background section of the two questionnaires was different; the employee questionnaire had a few more questions on the details of the Basic Health Insurance scheme. (See the appendix.)

A stratified quota random-sampling method was applied to select the two samples of respondents so as to aim at an even representation of the target populations. It enables equal numbers of respondents from chosen groups, but within each group, the random-sampling method is applied. The respective settings were used for setting the quota. Hospitals in China are now divided into three classes, as we mentioned earlier in chapter 3—levels one, two, and three; hospitals in level three have the best equipment and the most experienced and qualified medical staff. Standards at the other two levels move progressively downward. Employment units (the hiring units) are divided into three types by the nature of their ownership— first, state-owned enterprises; second, government bureaus and institutions; and third, private and foreign investment enterprises. Thirty units were selected randomly from the full list of 3,921 employment units that had participated in the city's Basic Health Insurance scheme at the time. On the hospital side, fifteen hospitals were also selected randomly from the total of 140 hospitals in Wuhan. Three hundred and five employees came variously from thirteen state-owned enterprises, ten government bureaus and institutions, and seven private and foreign investment enterprises; 302 patients came from fifteen hospitals, five from each level. All were interviewed in December 2003.

The Profile of the Two Samples

First we examine the profile of the respondents in table 5.1. Because of the lack of relevant population census data, we are not in a position to suggest that the two samples are representative either of the patient and working populations or of the general population of Wuhan. Nevertheless, a piece of finding is comforting.[8] The combined sample has a similar sex ratio to the general population of Wuhan—52.6 percent male and 47.4 percent female in our combined sample, while the general population of Wuhan had a ratio of 51.6 percent male and 48.4 percent female at the

Table 5.1 Demographic profile of respondents

	Employees	Patients	Overall	X_2
	% (N)	% (N)	% (N)	
Gender				
Male	54.1 (164)	51.0 (154)	52.6 (318)	.595
Female	45.9 (139)	49.0 (148)	47.4 (287)	
Total	100.0 (303)	100.0 (302)	100.0 (605)	
Age				
18–30	36.0 (109)	38.7 (117)	37.4 (226)	2.266
31–59	49.5 (150)	43.7 (132)	46.6 (282)	
60 or older	14.5 (44)	17.5 (53)	16.0 (97)	
Total	100.0 (303)	100.0 (302)	100.0 (605)	
Education				
Primary or below	3.4 (10)	8.4 (25)	5.9 (35)	28.831***
Secondary	26.9 (80)	43.1 (129)	35.1 (209)	
Tertiary or above	69.7 (207)	48.5 (145)	59.1 (352)	
Total	100.0 (297)	100.0 (299)	100.0 (596)	
Marital status				
Single	35.1 (104)	28.5 (85)	31.8 (189)	3.882
Married	61.5 (182)	66.1 (197)	63.8 (379)	
Other	3.4 (10)	5.4 (16)	4.4 (26)	
Total	100.0 (296)	100.0 (298)	100.0 (594)	
Ownership				
Stated-owned enterprises	63.1 (188)	44.1 (132)	53.6 (320)	21.528***
Other	36.9 (110)	55.9 (167)	46.4 (277)	
Total	100.0 (298)	100.0 (299)	100.0 (597)	
Personal income				
Below ¥1,000	48.1 (128)	18.4 (47)	33.5 (175)	69.933***
¥1,000–1,999	38.0 (101)	40.6 (104)	39.3 (205)	
¥2,000 or above	13.9 (37)	41.0 (105)	27.2 (142)	
Total	100.0 (266)	100.0 (256)	100.0 (522)	
Employment type				
Permanent worker	71.3 (204)			
Contracted worker	26.2 (75)			
Temporary worker	2.4 (7)			
Total	100.0 (286)			

*$p < 0.05$; ** $p < 0.01$; *** $p < 0.001$

end 2003. But, it is clear that our two respondent groups have a higher income than the average Wuhan residents. In terms of personal income, only 18.4 percent of the patient group earn less than 1,000 yuan, while nearly half of the employee group do so; similarly, the patient group is much richer. In comparison with Wuhan's average annual disposable income of 8,525 yuan for its residents in 2003, both groups are seemingly wealthier.

On age composition, it is interesting to note that the middle-aged people (31–59) are the largest group in all of the three samples—49.5 percent for the employee sample; 43.7 percent for the patient sample; and 46.6 percent for the combined one. We also have a patient sample with only 17.5 percent aged 60 years old and older (it is commonly supposed that the elderly always constitute the largest group of patients). The age distribution of the patient population is not available to us; the nearest comparative figures are the population distribution in Wuhan in 2003—when 0–14 year olds made up 22.1 percent, 15–64 70.4 percent, and 65 and older 7.5 percent.[9] Apparently, we have an older sample. On education, the combined sample and the individual ones are much more educated—69.7 percent of the employee sample, 48.5 percent of the patient sample, and 59.1 percent of the combined samples have at least tertiary education. Simply considering China as a developing country, the high level of education of our respondents suggests that they are the privileged few in society who can afford medical care. Despite the use of a stratified quoting sampling method, there is unfortunately more representation from state-owned enterprises, due to the difficulty of finding private and foreign investment enterprises for our samples. It is also a little unfortunate that the method of equal quota for each stratum was not strictly followed for practical reasons. Moreover, 71.3 percent of the employees are permanent workers; this reflects that enterprise reform has not yet reached full strength in Wuhan, as the aim of enterprise reform is to increase labor mobility by employing more contract-term employees as one of the key methods.

On the basis of this brief introduction, it is safe to suggest that the backgrounds of the sample populations are indicative of the nature of China's health insurance system. It serves the privileged few—our patients were seemingly able to pay their medical expenses because of their higher income levels; the employees were entitled to medical insurance as part of their employment package, even though their income was close to the average for Wuhan residents. If these privileged few, i.e., our respondents, were also worried about paying their medical expenses, it is very likely that the rest of the population are in a much worse position. We shall come back to this issue later when we examine the empirical evidence gathered from our two medium-scale social surveys.

Respondents' Experiences Regarding Basic Health Insurance

Wuhan follows the Zhenjiang's Three-Phase Passage Model (see chapter 3) for its Basic Health Insurance scheme. On the contribution side, individual employees pay 2 percent of their wages while employers contribute 8 percent of the monthly total wages to the scheme. The contribution rate of employers is a little higher than the mandatory 6 percent for employers as provided for in the 1998 State Council Decree, which lays down the principles and guidelines for the nation-wide medical insurance reform.

It is on the benefit side that the Three-Phase Passage Model derives its meaning. In Wuhan, the scheme works in the following three phases. First, insured employees have to pay their medical expenses from their personal accounts up to a threshold before they can start to claim from the socially pooled fund. The threshold amount is set at 10 percent of the average total wages of the previous year in Wuhan. This is the first tier, which aims to constrain demand. Second, when the initial self-paid amount is exhausted, employees begin to use the socially pooled fund up to a ceiling, which is set at four times the average annual wages for the previous year. Co-payment from personal accounts is required in this second phase, as another demand-constraining measure. Third, for treatment of serious illness, the amount of the ceiling for limiting reimbursement—that is, four times the city's annual average wage for the last year—may not be enough. Hence, there is a supplemental insurance, serious illness insurance, to pay for the treatment of serious illness. In Wuhan, the monthly individual payment for this supplemental serious illness insurance was set at 5 yuan and the maximum annual entitlement at 300,000 yuan. These amounts of contributions and benefits were set when Wuhan implemented its medical insurance scheme in 2001.

According to our survey findings, nearly half of the employees and only one quarter of the patients had experience using their personal medical accounts for co-paying medical expenses; the difference between two groups of respondents is statistically significant (table 5.2, statement 1). The difference may be due to the lower subscription rate of the patient group for basic health insurance.

We also asked the employee respondents whether they had experience using the socially pooled fund. Slightly less than one-fifth of them replied positively (table 5.2, statement 2). This may be due to the short history of Basic Health Insurance in Wuhan.

The employee respondents were also asked whether they have experience claiming insurance beyond the ceiling of the socially pooled fund. One-tenth of respondents from this group replied positively (table 5.2, statement 3). It seems to be a large figure, given the age composition of the employee respondent group (e.g., only 14.5 percent were sixty years old and older), and that the quite enormous amount of funds (i.e., four times the last year's annual average wage) had to be used before the respondents were able to claim beyond the ceiling. Two reasons may account for this large figure. First, medical expenses were really high. Second, two classical factors that fuel medical costs[10] might be at work in this case—moral hazard on the part of the patients and information asymmetry in the doctors' favor.

Table 5.2 Respondents' experiences with using medical insurance

	Employees	Patients	Overall	X^2
	% (N)	% (N)	% (N)	
1. Having experiences of using respondents' personal account for paying medical expenses.				
Have	49.6 (138)	25.0 (66)	37.6 (204)	35.036***
Haven't	50.4 (140)	75.0 (198)	62.4 (338)	
Total	100.0 (278)	100.0 (264)	100.0 (542)	
2. Having experiences of using social insurance fund for paying medical expenses.				
Have	17.9 (50)			
Haven't	82.1 (230)			
Total	100.0 (280)			
3. Having experiences of claiming insurance beyond the ceiling of the social insurance fund.				
Have	9.9 (25)			
Haven't	90.1 (227)			
Total	100.0 (252)			

*$p < 0.05$; ** $p < 0.01$; *** $p < 0.001$

Apart from the supplemental serious illness insurance, residents and employers (the hiring units) are also encouraged to purchase supplemental medical insurance. Labor unions and some other nongovernment organizations such as women's leagues are also involved in organizing supplemental insurance. This is different from the supplemental insurance against serious illness, which covers payments exceeding the ceiling in the Phase Model. This is used to subsidize people's personal medical accounts. Commercial insurance companies manage these supplemental insurance schemes; however, there is strong government involvement in the scheme for serious illness—here, the Social Insurance Center, the social-security-administration organ, represents the insured in signing the collective deal.

The findings in table 5.3 suggest that the idea of supplemental insurance for adding funding to personal medical accounts was not popular among our respondents. Three out of ten employee respondents, a significant minority and a quite high proportion, replied that their labor unions or other organizations had organized some voluntary supplemental insurance schemes for them; slightly less than one quarter of the same group of respondents suggested that they had purchased commercial medical insurance (table 5.3, statements 1 and 2). According to official statistics, 1.5 million people in Wuhan were subscribing to commercial medical insurance in May 2003. We should not assume that all of the commercial medical insurance subscribers are employees; it is likely that the noninsured, for example, the nonworking population such as children, youths, and housewives from the more wealthy families, are also subscribers. No wonder that a little more than the 1.3 million employees belong to the Basic Health Insurance at the same time. It can be argued that this is evidence that people need to purchase supplemental insurance given that out-of-pocket payments from personal funding are rising fast. Moreover, the contributions from both employees and employers to the Basic Health Insurance, i.e., roughly 10 percent of the total wages, are not sufficient to meet the sheer size of medical costs. A reference to the situation in Shanghai is indicative—the average medical consumption rate per person in 1999 there was more than 17 percent of the total wages.[11] However, it should be noted that Shanghai has the oldest urban population in China.

The Perceptions of the Underlying Features of the Basic Health Insurance

We would like to reveal the attitudes of respondents toward the health insurance reform in China by taking the case of our Wuhan respondents. Table 5.4 informs us about the respondents' views toward the underlying features of the Basic Health Insurance. It seems that the mix of a socially pooled fund for redistribution and a personal savings account for personal accumulation is acceptable to most of the employee respondents—only a quarter of them disagreed with the arrangement, while half of them took a positive view (table 5.4, statement 1). Moreover, when the employee respondents were asked which of the funds should be allocated more of the contributions, slightly more favored personal accounts than the socially pooled fund (52.4 percent versus 47.6 percent) (table 5.4, statement 2).

The major item of reform in medical insurance is the requirement of individual co-payments for health care protection, a feature that was unheard of in the pre-reform era. Nearly two-thirds of employee respondents (73.5 percent) and four-fifths of patient respondents (79.8 percent) agreed that it is reasonable for individuals to bear part of their medical expenses (table 5.4, statement 3). There is no statistical difference between the two samples. Coupled with the response pattern of the previous statement about the divide on the allocation of the contribution, these response patterns are remarkable,

Table 5.3 Employees' participation in supplemental health insurance

	%	(N)
1. Labor unions or other organizations had organized some voluntary supplemental insurance schemes.		
Yes	29.3	(78)
No	70.7	(188)
Total	100.0	(266)
2. Have purchased commercial medical insurance.		
Have	23.1	(65)
Haven't	76.9	(216)
Total	100.0	(281)

Table 5.4 Respondents' views toward the main features of the Basic Health Insurance

	Employees		Patients		Overall		X^2
	%	(N)	%	(N)	%	(N)	
1. The arrangement of a social insurance fund and personal account is reasonable.							
Agree/Strongly agree	51.1	(116)					
Half-half	23.4	(53)					
Disagree/Strongly disagree	25.5	(58)					
Total	100.0	(227)					
2. Which fund should be allocated more?							
Social insurance fund	47.6	(88)					
Personal account	52.4	(97)					
Total	100.0	(185)					
3. It is reasonable for an individual to bear part of his or her medical expenses.							
Agree/Strongly agree	73.5	(216)	79.8	(229)	76.6	(445)	3.246
Half-half	15.3	(45)	11.5	(33)	13.4	(78)	
Disagree/Strongly disagree	11.2	(33)	8.7	(25)	10.0	(58)	
Total	100.0	(294)	100.0	(287)	100.0	(581)	

$*p < 0.05$; $**p < 0.01$; $***p < 0.001$

suggesting that, after two decades of economic reform, the Chinese have accepted the main underlying principle of the market mechanism, i.e., individual responsibility for one's own welfare. Clearly, their earlier experiences of similar arrangements in the area of old-age pensions have contributed to the high acceptance rates here.

The Perceptions of Reform of Hospitals

We confine our discussion of the reform of medical establishments to hospitals. Since the 1980s, government funding to hospitals has been declining, as we mentioned in chapter 2. According to China's official statistics, the government health budget was 36.2 percent of total health sector expenditure in 1980, 25 percent in 1990, and only 17 percent in 1995.[12] We shall discuss this point later in chapter 6, but a reasonable guess is that the decline in the government health budget as a percentage of total health expenditure demonstrates that the basic strategy of decentralizing both the financing and administration of health care to hospitals has been an effective policy from the standpoint of controlling the government's financial commitments. Since 1980, health care has been changing from a social welfare to a fee-for-service system.[13]

In the absence of sufficient funding from the government, hospitals have to rely on fee charges and drug sales as the main sources of revenue. Many reforms designed to improve the mechanisms of competition are being introduced to hospitals, the objectives being to reduce medical costs and to increase choice for patients. For example, employees are now able to choose health care providers within their locality from a certified catalog list. Another example of these reform initiatives is the requirement for doctors to prescribe drugs from a certified list. The latest measure adopted by many local medical insurance centers is to fix a gross amount for the payment to the contracted hospitals.[14] This step will reduce the risk for medical insurance centers. However, this risk reduction exercise may result in a trade-off in which health care quality could well be the loser.

Against these backgrounds, we would like to know, from the perception of stakeholders, whether and how far hospital reforms succeed in reducing abuses and costs and increasing patient choices.

Nearly four out of five respondents from both the employee and patient groups agreed with the statement that health care reform can reduce patients' abuse of health services, such as treating minor illnesses as serious ones (table 5.5, statement 1). No statistical significance is found between the two groups. However, many more patients than employees agree that health care reform can reduce doctors' intentional prescription of expensive drugs—74.6 percent of patients as against 63.7 of employees; and there is statistical significance between the two groups (table 5.5, statement 2). Seemingly, reform initiatives in hospitals can change both patients' and doctors' behavior in regard to abuses, resulting in cost reductions.

Evidently, more patients than employees are positive about one effect of hospital

Table 5.5 Respondents' views of the effects of reform initiatives on hospitals

	Employees		Patients		Overall		X^2
	%	(N)	%	(N)	%	(N)	
1. Health care reforms can reduce a patient's abuse of health service, such as treating minor illness as serious illness.							
Agree/Strongly agree	72.9	(255)	77.1	(216)	78.2	(441)	.361
Half-half	9.5	(27)	10.4	(29)	9.9	(56)	
Disagree/Strongly disagree	11.3	(32)	12.5	(35)	11.9	(67)	
Total	100.0	(284)	100.0	(280)	100.0	(564)	
2. Health care reform can reduce a doctor's intentional prescription of expensive drugs.							
Agree/Strongly agree	63.7	(179)	74.6	(209)	69.2	(399)	8.954*
Half-half	14.9	(42)	12.5	(35)	13.7	(77)	
Disagree/Strongly disagree	21.4	(60)	12.9	(36)	17.1	(96)	
Total	100.0	(281)	100.0	(280)	100.0	(561)	
3. Now consulting doctors is more convenient than it was before.							
Agree/Strongly agree	64.4	(181)	79.0	(229)	71.8	(410)	15.354***
Half-half	16.7	(47)	11.0	(32)	13.8	(79)	
Disagree/Strongly disagree	18.9	(53)	10.0	(29)	14.4	(82)	
Total	100.0	(281)	100.0	(290)	100.0	(571)	
4. Now patients have more choices of doctors and hospitals than they had before.							
Agree/Strongly agree	74.2	(213)	58.7	(245)	79.9	(458)	12.003**
Half-half	11.1	(32)	7.0	(20)	9.1	(52)	
Disagree/Strongly disagree	14.6	(42)	7.3	(21)	11.0	(63)	
Total	100.0	(287)	100.0	(286)	100.0	(573)	
5. Now service quality provided by doctors and hospitals is better than it was before.							
Agree/Strongly agree	47.3	(132)	62.6	(179)	55.0	(311)	13.915**
Half-half	27.2	(76)	17.5	(50)	22.3	(126)	
Disagree/Strongly disagree	25.4	(71)	19.9	(57)	22.7	(128)	
Total	100.0	(279)	100.0	(286)	100.0	(565)	

*$p < 0.05$; ** $p < 0.01$; *** $p < 0.001$

reform—79 percent of the former and 64.4 percent of the latter now find it more convenient to consult doctors than it was before the health care reform (table 5.5, statement 3). The difference between the two groups is statistically significant. But the absolute values of both groups are high. In the same vein, both groups are also happy about having greater choice of doctors and hospitals now than before the health care reform—74.2 percent of the employee respondents and 85.7 percent of the patient respondents; the difference is also statistically significant (table 5.5, statement 4). It is clear, from the perceptions of two important stakeholders, that hospital reforms have improved substantially the delivery quality of medical services. Nevertheless, when the substantive question on service quality is asked, the agreement ratios are less favorable as compared with those of the last two statements—only less than half of the employee respondents and about two-thirds of the patient respondents agree that the quality of services provided by doctors and hospitals is now better than it was before the health care reform; there is statistical significance between the two groups (table 5.5, statement 5).

In general, hospital reforms have received very positive responses from two key stakeholders, employees and patients. The patient respondents are even more positive than the employee respondents. It is suggested that the difference between them is likely due to the personal experiences of the former. In light of this, further progress in the hospital reforms would yield further positive results.

The Perceptions of the Reform of the Medicine Production and Circulation System

The reform of the medicine production and circulation system is designed to control the cost of medicines, the quality of medicines, and the qualifications of pharmacists. We focus our study more on the first part of the objective—that is, on whether cost control is successful—on the basis of the findings of the perceptions of the two respondent samples. Nevertheless, the control of costs may have an impact on the quality of medicines available to patients, and this is an equity issue. From the viewpoint of the regulating authorities, the primary concern is the quality of medicine itself, but whether quality medicine is accessible to all is not their key concern at the operational level. It is found that only one-third of the employee respondents, but nearly half of the patient respondents, agree with the statement that "the current limit on reimbursement of medicine is reasonable" (table 5.6, statement 1). There is statistical significance between the two groups. Evidently, the cost-containing method is more effective for the patients than for the employees. In practice, the reimbursement limit of medicine does deprive many patients of quality medicines for treatment, and many others have to pay out of their own pockets for medicines not in the catalog but endorsed by the medical insurance centers.

A further cost-containment measure is the setting of uniform prices for drugs.

Table 5.6 Respondents' views toward the control of the costs of medicine

	Employees		Patients		Overall		X^2
	%	(N)	%	(N)	%	(N)	
1. The current limit on the reimbursement of medicine is reasonable.							
Agree/Strongly agree	32.6	(88)	46.1	(119)	39.2	(207)	10.503**
Half-half	32.6	(88)	27.9	(72)	30.3	(160)	
Disagree/Strongly disagree	34.8	(94)	26.0	(67)	30.5	(161)	
Total	100.0	(270)	100.0	(258)	100.0	(528)	
2. The proportion of drug cost to medical consultation:							
Very high/High	87.9	(155)	71.3	(209)	79.4	(455)	25.561***
Average	11.4	(32)	24.2	(71)	18.0	(103)	
Low/Very low	.7	(2)	4.4	(13)	2.6	(15)	
Total	100.0	(280)	100.0	(293)	100.0	(573)	
3. Most cost-effective place to purchase drugs:							
Hospitals/Clinics	5.3	(15)	9.2	(24)	7.1	(39)	8.006*
Pharmacies	81.7	(232)	77.1	(202)	79.5	(434)	
Units' clinics	2.1	(6)	5.3	(14)	3.7	(20)	
Others	10.9	(31)	8.4	(22)	9.7	(53)	
Total	100.0	(284)	100.0	(262)	100.0	(546)	
4. The usual place to purchase drugs after medical consultation in hospitals and clinics:							
Hospitals/Clinics	42.3	(127)	50.3	(150)	46.3	(277)	5.683
Pharmacies	46.7	(140)	42.3	(126)	44.5	(266)	
Units' clinics	9.0	(27)	6.7	(20)	7.9	(47)	
Others	2.0	(6)	.7	(2)	1.3	(8)	
Total	100.0	(300)	100.0	(298)	100.0	(598)	

*$p < 0.05$; ** $p < 0.01$; *** $p < 0.001$

The effective application of this measure depends not only on the regulation of the production and retailing of medicines but even more on the regulation of sales of drugs by doctors and hospitals. Since hospitals have to rely on the sale of medicine as a major source of revenue, it is in the interest of doctors and hospitals to sell medicine directly to patients. Due to the limited public funding, hospitals are allowed to take a 15 percent profit margin on sales of drugs to compensate them for insufficient funding. This gives rise to what looks like a paradoxical situation: An excessively rigorous regulatory regime would be against the interests of the government, because if hospitals cannot obtain sufficient revenue from selling drugs, they will be forced to turn to the government for assistance. This points to a structural source of problems in containing the cost of medicines in China.

We now come to examine the outcome of the reform initiatives for cost-containment in the medicine production and circulation system. In the perception of the respondents, drug costs are still very high. In total, 87.9 percent of the employee respondents and 71.3 percent of the patient respondents agree that the proportion of drug costs to the costs of medical consultation is, respectively, "very high" and "high" (table 5.6, statement 2). The difference between the two groups is statistically significant. A reasonable guess is that because patients make more use of medicines, they are more accustomed to the high cost. However, this finding suggests that the reform initiatives aimed at controlling the cost of drugs have not been successful. Perhaps the vested interests of doctors and hospitals are at the root of this. This conclusion is supported by the following responses to the two questions we posed to the respondents, regarding their knowledge of where they could purchase cheaper drugs and where they usually conduct the purchase.

If the consumer is the best judge, respondents should be smart enough to know where they can purchase cheaper drugs. In accordance with our findings, the pharmacy was clearly the preferred choice—77.1 percent of patient respondents and 81.7 percent of employee respondents selected this as the favored choice; only 9.2 percent of the former and 5.3 percent of the latter took hospitals and clinics as the cheaper alternative (table 5.6, statement 3). However, only 42.3 percent of the patient respondents and 46.7 percent of the employee respondents purchased their drugs in pharmacies as their usual source after medical consultation in hospitals and clinics (table 5.6, statement 4). There is no statistical significance between the two groups. Convenience is the most likely explanation. Given that drug costs are considered very high, it is safe to assume that people would not mind going to pharmacies for bargain prices. Unfortunately, we did not ask for an explanation for this unusual phenomenon, which is clearly advantageous to doctors and hospitals. Our earlier discussion on the high drug cost in chapter 3 should be helpful.

To conclude, respondents had mixed feelings about the current limit on the reimbursement of their spending on medicines; most of them, especially the employee respondents, regarded drug costs to be high, to varying extents. Despite higher prices, many of them usually purchased drugs in hospitals. As was mentioned in the previous section, a list of twenty pharmacies or designated drug retailors in Wuhan, in the initial phase, were authorized to sell medicines to the insured under the Basic Health Insurance. However, on the basis of these findings, one may doubt the effectiveness of the reform initiatives on the control of the cost of medicines.

From Policy Issues to Underlying Ideologies

The issues of chief concern in health care policy are equity, efficiency, and affordability.[15] We define the ideologies corresponding to these issues as those related to welfarism, neo-liberalism, and social developmentalism, as suggested in the earlier part of this book. We leave out welfare pluralism here, not because it is not important in the Chinese context, but because in this section we confine ourselves to exploring the previous three issues, which essentially cluster around the role of the state in health care protection. Welfare pluralism is more concerned with the ways in which service provision is organized to avoid bureaucracy and inefficiency.

Welfarism can be understood as the principal tenet underpinning the role of the state in health care. Welfarism represents the view that it is the state and not the individual who should bear the primary responsibility for health care. In the Chinese context, the old system of health care enabled urban employees in government offices, state-owned enterprises, and some collective enterprises to enjoy free or cheap medical services while employees of the newly emerging foreign and private enterprises were not given the necessary protection. This system had to be reformed to enhance labor mobility and reduce production costs.[16] Both are efficiency issues.

The opposing ideology to welfarism is neo-liberalism, which regards the market mechanism as the panacea for the ills associated with welfarism. Neo-liberalism regards privatization as the principal step in dismantling welfarism. In the Chinese case, what one sees is not exactly the complete elimination of welfarism coupled with a comprehensive move toward privatization. The Chinese emphasis is on individual responsibility in health care protection rather than on complete privatization. Even at that, the shift toward individual responsibility in China is partial only. Responsibility is shared between the individual and the state, as exemplified in the mixed model of the socially pooled fund and personal medical accounts in the Basic Health Insurance scheme.

Apparently, health care reform in China has been a gradual process carried out in piecemeal steps. In the course of this gradual process, it is important to make a cross-sectional assessment to see whether there is a shift, from the perceptions of our respondents, in terms of the responsibility for health care. It is presumed that through social surveys, the policy issues of equity and efficiency can be examined.

The ideology of social developmentalism is also added in our study. In essence, it is about the role of the state in harmonizing social and economic development.[17] Social developmentalism is especially relevant to the Chinese case because in the wake of health care reform, numerous problems have cropped up: the growing inequalities in the access to health services, the increases in the cost of medical care and medicine, and the deterioration of preventive health services in the rural areas. In the end, we are trying to see whether equitable and affordable health care is generally followed by economic growth—more specifically, whether the issue of a fine balance between the need for health care protection and the need for economic development is properly addressed, from the perceptions of the two stakeholder groups in our surveys.

The Perceptions of Responsibility in Health Care

Table 5.7 illustrates whether there is a shift in responsibility as reflected from the perceptions of the respondents. It is assumed that the responsibility structure for health care should reflect the profile of the ideologies underpinning health care, as perceived from the two stakeholders' groups.

An overwhelming majority of the two respondent groups regard the government or the employment units as having the responsibility for assisting those who are unable to pay their medical fees: 83.2 percent of the employee respondents and 88.2 percent of the patient respondents (table 5.7, statement 1). No statistical significance is detected between the two groups. A collective responsibility is perceived, especially in the case of low-income people. The present policy arrangements, in which the major financial responsibilities are devolved to the employment units and from the employment units to individual employees, are not supported by either of the respondent groups. Apparently, the government is perceived as having the final responsibility in health care protection. In the same vein, a slightly larger number of respondents from both groups disagreed with the statement that "the government has no responsibility to provide basic health care to all"—around nine out of ten in both groups. This can be interpreted as a strong endorsement of the ideology of welfarism (table 5.7, statement 2). As with the first statement, no statistical significance is found between the two groups. This statement received a greater endorsement. Hence, it can be suggested that the traditional belief in social protection underpinning the command economy is still pretty much alive among the two respondent groups. These findings are in line with an earlier survey in 1996 in Shanghai, which also identified a strong welfarist orientation of respondents in health care protection. About three quarters of the Shanghai respondents endorsed the following statement—"Government should be responsible for one's medical expenses."[18] It is important to note that the same respondent group in Shanghai had also seen major improvements in living standards and employment conditions due to economic reform. In other words, economic reform does not remove the traditional belief in the state's role in health care protection.

Table 5.7 Respondents' perceptions of responsibility in health care

	Employees		Patients		Overall		X^2
	%	(N)	%	(N)	%	(N)	
1. Those who are not able to pay for medical fees should be assisted by the government or the employment unit							
Agree/Strongly agree	83.2	(247)	88.2	(262)	85.7	(509)	4.626
Half-half	8.8	(26)	7.7	(23)	8.2	(49)	
Disagree/Strongly disagree	8.1	(24)	4.0	(12)	6.1	(36)	
Total	100.0	(297)	100.0	(297)	100.0	(594)	
2. The government has no responsibility to provide basic health care to all.							
Agree/Strongly agree	5.4	(16)	8.3	(24)	6.8	(40)	1.889
Half-half	3.1	(9)	2.8	(8)	2.9	(17)	
Disagree/Strongly disagree	91.5	(270)	89.0	(258)	90.3	(528)	
Total	100.0	(295)	100.0	(290)	100.0	(585)	
3. It is reasonable to treat urban and rural residents differently in terms of health care benefits.							
Agree/Strongly agree	24.3	(68)	28.1	(77)	26.2	(145)	5.918
Half-half	18.6	(52)	11.3	(31)	15.0	(83)	
Disagree/Strongly disagree	57.1	(160)	60.6	(166)	58.8	(326)	
Total	100.0	(280)	100.0	(274)	100.0	(554)	
4. One should not be entitled to health care protection if one does not pay for medical insurance.							
Agree/Strongly agree	47.0	(134)	39.9	(115)	43.5	(249)	3.775
Half-half	17.2	(49)	16.7	(48)	16.9	(97)	
Disagree/Strongly disagree	35.8	(102)	43.4	(125)	39.6	(227)	
Total	100.0	(285)	100.0	(288)	100.0	(573)	
5. Medical expenses are the primary responsibility of individuals, employment units, or the government.							
Individual	13.1	(33)	14.6	(36)	13.9	(69)	0.370
Employment units	34.1	(86)	32.1	(79)	33.1	(165)	
Government	52.8	(133)	53.3	(131)	53.0	(264)	
Total	100.0	(252)	100.0	(246)	100.0	(498)	
6. Which one of the following should be responsible for medical expenses above the ceiling if patients do not have medical insurance for serious illness?							
Individual	24.4	(45)	17.0	(31)	20.7	(76)	3.443
Employment units	22.0	(41)	20.9	(38)	21.5	(79)	
Government	53.8	(100)	62.1	(113)	57.9	(213)	
Total	100.0	(186)	100.0	(182)	100.0	(368)	

*$p < 0.05$; ** $p < 0.01$; *** $p < 0.001$

With reference to the dual treatment of urban and rural residents in China's health care system, around six out of ten from both groups disagreed to the statement that "it is reasonable to treat urban and rural residents differently in terms of health care benefits" (table 5.7, statement 3). The proportions adopting a social equity stance in this case dropped a little as compared with the previous two sets of responses, but they remained more than a simple majority. In this last instance, the appeal of welfarism in health care clearly extends to the rural residents. However, when dealing with the practical level, the ideological stance was put aside for a while. Slightly less than half of the employee respondents and two-fifths of the patient respondents supported the statement that "one should not be entitled to health care protection if one does not pay for medical insurance" (table 5.7, statement 4). No statistical significance is found between the two groups. A sense of pragmatism is thus found alongside the ideology of welfarism. Perhaps this can be regarded as forming the foundation for social developmentalism.

Two further statements are used to test whether there has been a shift in the policy assumption toward more individual responsibility in health care. The response patterns seem to be negative. Still slightly more than half of both respondent groups regard the government as having "the primary responsibility for medical expenses," another one-third in both groups saw the employment units as primarily responsible, and the remaining 13.1 percent of the employee group and 14.6 percent of the patient group favored individual responsibility (table 5.7, statement 5). A similar pattern is revealed when we asked about the medical expenses above the ceiling in the Three-Phase Passage Model in the case where the patient did not have medical insurance for serious illness. A little more than half of the employee group and three-fifths of the patient group viewed the government as holding the responsibility; slightly more than one-fifth of both groups endorsed the employment units. However, more of the employee group—24.2 percent—and 17 percent of the patient group perceived patients and their families as having the responsibility for expenses beyond the ceiling (table 5.7, statement 6). No statistical significance between both groups on statements 5 and 6 was found.

The Perceptions of Out-of-Pocket Payments

Despite the strong preference for welfarism, underpinned by the policy assumption of collective responsibility, and state responsibility in particular, the respondents would not necessarily choose policy options that reflect individual responsibility for health care arrangements beyond basic levels. Table 5.8 shows statements along these lines to test whether the aforementioned assumption is reasonable. A mixed response pattern is discerned (see table 5.8). The two groups take a similar

Table 5.8 Respondents' views of out-of-pocket payment for health care

	Employees		Patients		Overall		X^2
	%	(N)	%	(N)	%	(N)	
1. Out-of-pocket payment for expert consultation is right.							
Agree/Strongly agree	39.4	(114)	42.3	(124)	40.9	(238)	5.120
Half-half	18.7	(54)	24.2	(71)	21.5	(125)	
Disagree/Strongly disagree	41.9	(121)	33.4	(98)	37.6	(219)	
Total	100.0	(289)	100.0	(293)	100.0	(582)	
2. Out-of-pocket payment for high-tech medical equipment is right.							
Agree/Strongly agree	28.3	(81)	29.8	(86)	29.0	(167)	.167
Half-half	21.7	(62)	20.8	(60)	21.2	(122)	
Disagree/Strongly disagree	50.0	(143)	49.5	(143)	49.7	(286)	
Total	100.0	(286)	100.0	(289)	100.0	(575)	
3. Out-of-pocket payment for high-quality medicines is right.							
Agree/Strongly agree	43.4	(124)	45.0	(130)	44.2	(254)	.363
Half-half	21.0	(60)	19.0	(55)	20.0	(115)	
Disagree/Strongly disagree	35.7	(102)	36.0	(104)	35.8	(206)	
Total	100.0	(286)	100.0	(289)	100.0	(575)	
4. Out-of-pocket payment for staying at high-class wards is right.							
Agree/Strongly agree	63.4	(184)	64.7	(189)	64.1	(373)	.155
Half-half	16.9	(49)	15.8	(46)	16.3	(95)	
Disagree/Strongly disagree	19.7	(57)	19.5	(57)	19.6	(114)	
Total	100.0	(290)	100.0	(292)	100.0	(582)	

*$p < 0.05$; ** $p < 0.01$; *** $p < 0.001$

view on out-of-pocket payments for expert consultations—around two-fifths of both employee and patient groups agree with the statement, while two-fifths of the employee group and one-third of the patient group endorse the opposite view (table 5.8, statement 1). No statistical significance is found between the two groups.

On out-of-pocket payments for high-technology medical equipment, half of the respondents from both groups feel it is not right for individuals to bear the responsibility; around one-third of respondents from both groups endorse the opposite statement (table 5.8, statement 2). It is also found that there is no statistical significance between the two groups. A slightly different pattern is discerned on out-of-pocket payments for high-quality medicines—more than 43.4 percent of the employee group and 45 percent of the patient group think that it is right to place the responsibility of this aspect on individuals, while 35.7 percent of the former and 36 percent of the latter disagree (table 5.8, statement 3). Furthermore, the last statement on out-of-pocket payments, for staying in high-class wards, receive the strongest approval rates from both groups of respondents—nearly two-thirds from each group endorse it (table 5.8, statement 4). There is no statistical significance between the two groups of respondents on both statements.

In sum, the response patterns on out-of-pocket payment are rather mixed—they differ from item to item; however, one clear indicator is apparent—respondents perceive different extents of individual responsibility for the different forms of medical treatment beyond basic levels. It can also be inferred that the respondents are moderate; they do not support welfarism beyond basic levels. Two factors may explain this attitude: First, China is still a developing country despite its immediate past as a command economy that provided comprehensive employment-based welfare, or *workfare,* through the work entities (*danwei*);[19] second, Chinese culture includes a strong ethos of self-reliance, and welfare is seen as an expression of benevolence rather than as a matter of rights.[20] In policy terms, coupled with the set of responses in table 5.7, this means that the state has responsibility for health care for all, but it does not mean that people do not need to pay for it. Individual responsibility has a central place in health care reform, and this explains the endorsement by patients of the privatization strategy underpinning the ideology of neo-liberalism.

The Perceptions of the Relationship Between Economic Development and Health Care

We now consider whether the findings of the two social surveys support any linkage between health care protection and the need for economic development. The first statement in table 5.9 suggests that an overwhelming majority of the respondents from both groups disagree that "the primary role of the government is economic development and not welfare improvement"—84.6 percent of the employee group and 86.7 percent of the patient group; there is no difference in terms of statistical significance between the two groups. In other words, the respondents do not see a trade-off between economic development and welfare development. Welfare development has a life of its own. Does this response pattern reflect an endorsement of social developmentalism? The following survey findings might provide us with some pointers.

It can be assumed that if there is a fine balance between economic growth and health care protection, respondents will be inclined to agree more with statements about the affordability of medical treatments. This is not the case in the response patterns for the following two statements. Nearly three quarters of respondents from both groups agree, to different extents, that "medical expenses exceed what our country can afford under the current economic condition" (table 5.9, statement 2). No statistical significance between the two groups is detected. Implicitly, from the perceptions of the respondents, medical expenses are costly in relation to China's level of economic prosperity. In a related question, somewhat more respondents from both groups, 86.1 percent of the employee respondents and

Table 5.9 Respondents' perceptions of economic development and health care

	Employees		Patients		Overall		X_2
	%	(N)	%	(N)	%	(N)	
1. The primary role of the government is economic development and not welfare improvement.							
Agree/Strongly agree	11.3	(33)	8.5	(25)	9.9	(58)	1.353
Half-half	4.1	(12)	4.8	(14)	4.4	(26)	
Disagree/Strongly disagree	84.6	(247)	86.7	(254)	85.6	(501)	
Total	100.0	(292)	100.0	(293)	100.0	(585)	
2. Medical expenses exceed what our country can afford under the current economic condition.							
Agree/Strongly agree	73.5	(202)	75.4	(205)	74.4	(407)	.908
Half-half	11.3	(31)	8.8	(24)	10.1	(55)	
Disagree/Strongly disagree	15.3	(42)	15.8	(43)	15.5	(85)	
Total	100.0	(275)	100.0	(272)	100.0	(547)	
3. The current medical examination and treatment expenses exceed what the general public can afford.							
Agree/Strongly agree	86.1	(255)	84.7	(243)	85.4	(498)	1.188
Half-half	6.4	(19)	8.7	(25)	7.5	(44)	
Disagree/Strongly disagree	7.4	(22)	6.6	(19)	7.0	(41)	
Total	100.0	(296)	100.0	(287)	100.0	(583)	

$*p < 0.05$; $**p < 0.01$; $***p < 0.001$

84.7 percent of the patient respondents, agree that "the current medical examination and treatment expenses exceed what the general public can afford" (table 5.9, statement 3). Here also, there is no statistical significance between the two groups. Taking all of these responses together as evidence, there has not been an appropriate balance, in the perceptions of the respondents, between economic growth and health care protection. The findings do not tell us where the right balance lies; however, it is clear that, at present, affordability is a critical and major issue in the perception of the respondents. On the basis of this discussion, it can be inferred that the respondents generally endorse the principal tenet of social developmentalism and that the state has a role in harmonizing social and economic development. They think that the present model for the funding of medical services is not right because it exceeds what the economy and the general public can afford.

Litmus Test of the Support for Health Care Reform

Here, in table 5.10, we examine the overall question of whether it is necessary to start health care reform despite the problems associated with it, such as affordability and equity. This question serves as a litmus test of the support for health care reform. Moreover, as is stated at the beginning of this chapter, the overall objective of the health care reform in China is to provide better-quality medical services at relatively cheap costs to satisfy the basic medical needs of the ordinary people. At this point in the course of health care reform, how the two key stakeholders—the patients and employees who form the two respondent groups—regard the essential question of health care affordability in the Wuhan context helps us toward an understanding of the progress and problems of health care reform in the country as a whole.

More than eight out of ten respondents from both groups agree, to different extents, that the health care system must be changed (table 5.10, statement 1). No statistical significance is detected between the two groups. Apparently, health care reform is generally welcome, at least as far as the two key stakeholders in our surveys are concerned. In other words, health care reform is supported in principle. We then come to the question whether people believe that they also benefit from health care reform. Nearly two-thirds of the patient respondents, but slightly more than half of the employee respondents, agree to different extent that the current health care protection in Wuhan is better than that before economic reform (table 5.10, statement 2). More patients than employees agree; and the difference between the two groups is statistically significant. The approval rates of the last statement are substantially smaller than those of the statement about the necessity of change in the health care system. The cross-reference of the response patterns in table 5.5 should be useful here—respondents are generally

Table 5.10 Respondents' perceptions of overall outcome of health care reform

	Employees		Patients		Overall		X^2
	%	(N)	%	(N)	%	(N)	
1. Health care system must be changed.							
Agree/Strongly agree	81.8	(229)	81.3	(226)	81.5	(455)	4.377
Half-half	8.9	(25)	12.9	(36)	10.9	(61)	
Disagree/Strongly disagree	9.3	(26)	5.8	(16)	7.5	(42)	
Total	100	(280)	100	(278)	100	(558)	
2. The current health care protection in Wuhan is better than that before the economic reform.							
Agree/Strongly agree	53.5	(147)	64.3	(171)	58.8	(318)	6.563*
Half-half	20.0	(55)	15.0	(40)	17.6	(95)	
Disagree/Strongly disagree	26.5	(73)	20.7	(55)	23.7	(128)	
Total	100	(275)	100	(266)	100	(541)	
3. The current individual responsibility on medical expenses is:							
Too heavy	62.8	(503)	63.0	(160)	62.9	(310)	.420
Just fine	34.3	(82)	33.1	(84)	33.7	(166)	
Care bear more	2.9	(7)	3.9	(10)	3.4	(17)	
Total	100	(239)	100	(254)	100	(493)	
4. It is common that people are afraid of seeking medical consultation when they are ill in Wuhan.							
Agree/Strongly agree	68.2	(193)	61.7	(177)	64.9	(370)	4.142
Half-half	19.8	(56)	20.6	(59)	20.2	(115)	
Disagree/Strongly disagree	12.0	(34)	17.8	(51)	14.9	(85)	
Total	100	(283)	100	(287)	100	(570)	
5. I worry about medical expenses in the case of serious illness.							
Worry/Worry a lot	93.5	(275)	86.6	(253)	90.1	(529)	9.094*
Half-half	3.7	(11)	5.5	(16)	4.6	(27)	
Not worry/Completely not worry	2.7	(8)	7.9	(23)	5.3	(31)	
Total	100	(294)	100	(292)	100	(586)	
6. Worry about health care protection after retirement.							
Worry/Worry a lot	85.5	(248)			85.5	(248)	
Half-half	8.3	(24)			8.3	(24)	
Not worry/Completely not worry	6.2	(18)			6.2	(18)	
Total	100	(290)			100	(290)	
7. Don't worry about Wuhan's future health care protection.							
Agree/Strongly agree	20.2	(56)	31.0	(85)	25.6	(141)	8.544*
Half-half	18.8	(52)	15.3	(42)	17.1	(94)	
Disagree/Strongly disagree	61.0	(169)	53.6	(147)	57.4	(316)	
Total	100	(277)	100	(274)	100	(551)	

*$p < 0.05$; ** $p < 0.01$; *** $p < 0.001$

satisfied with the immediate effects of the reform initiatives on hospitals, such as the reduction of patients' and doctors' abuses of the health care system.

However, the overwhelming acceptance of the need for reform and the moderate benefits reportedly gained from reform do not necessarily indicate that respondents are satisfied that the overall objective of health care reform in China—the provision of better-quality medical services at relatively cheap costs—has been achieved. Note that these two respondent groups are the privileged few, as we have explained earlier. If these respondents express worries about the affordability of medical expenses, then one may doubt whether the objective of health care reform is achieved for the population as a whole.

As discussed earlier, the main thrust of health care reform is a policy shift, from the emphasis on collective responsibility, and state responsibility in particular, to one that includes individual responsibility in health care protection. Judging from the response patterns in table 5.7, the reform has not been successful. This begs the question how the respondents feel about the newly assigned individual responsibility in terms of medical expenses, and this can be seen as a litmus test for the affordability question in the perspective of the respondents. Perhaps people may exaggerate the burden of their newfound responsibility for health care. In the old systems of the publicly funded General Insurance and employer-funded Labor Insurance, employees of government bureaus and state-owned enterprises *basically* enjoyed free medicine, so that even a slight increase from that position might be regarded as too heavy. It is, of course, difficult to judge whether the increase has been only a slight increase or whether in fact it has been a substantial, even an unbearable one. It is necessary to consider these concerns when examining the responses.

Apparently, about two-thirds of both respondent groups consider that the levels of responsibility for medical expenses currently being placed on individuals are too heavy; only about one-third of both respondent groups replied that their share is acceptable; and only a small proportion feel that they could bear more (table 5.10, statement 3). No statistical significant difference is found between the two respondent groups. It is necessary to look for more clues of whether the new levels of individual responsibility for health care costs are really too heavy.

The litmus test is whether people are afraid of seeking medical consultation when they are ill in Wuhan. Nearly seven out of ten employee respondents and nearly six out of ten patient respondents agree, to varying extents, that they are (table 10, statement 4). No statistical difference is found between the two respondent groups. Although these response sizes amount to little more than a simple majority and fall short of being an overwhelming majority (e.g., over three quarters), it is fair to say that not consulting doctors was a common phenomenon in Wuhan when our surveys were conducted in late 2003, two years after the Basic Health Insurance was initiated. This is indeed a worrying phenomenon in terms of health care protection.

An overwhelming majority of respondents in both groups also worry about medical expenses in case of serious illness: 93.5 percent of the employee respondents and 86.6 percent of the patient respondents, to different extents (table 5.10, statement 5). There is a statistical significance between the two groups; perhaps employee respondents have less income than the patient respondents. This does not mean that the patient respondents do not worry about medical expenses in case of serious illness. The employee respondents also worry about health care protection after their retirement: 85.5 percent of them have this worry (table 5.10, statement 6). This statement was not put to the patient respondents because some of them were not in the labor market. The last statement asks respondents about their confidence in Wuhan's future health care protection; only one-fifth of the employee respondents and three-tenths of the patient respondents do not worry about Wuhan's future health care protection; this is indeed not an optimistic response pattern (table 5.10, statement 7). More employees than patients worry about Wuhan's future health care; the difference is statistically significant. In general, employee respondents worry more about their health care than their patient counterparts in as much as they perceive less improvement in health care protection as compared with the pre-economic reform era, expect less help with medical expenses for serious illness treatment, and see a less hopeful future for Wuhan's health care protection (table 5.10, statements 2, 5, and 7). In policy terms, it can be inferred that the employee population, especially those in the state-owned enterprises, are the losers in the course of economic reform in general and health care reform in particular. The transition to a market economy has definitely meant a redistribution of benefits and burdens among different socioeconomic groups.

To conclude, respondents are generally in favor of health care reform; they feel that there has been improvement as compared with the pre-economic reform period. However, the general endorsement of health care reform does not mean the respondents are equally supportive on the key question about the affordability of health care—medical expenses, especially for serious illness, are too heavy a burden on them; a substantial majority are afraid of seeking medical consultation when they are ill in Wuhan. Hence, the shift toward more individual responsibility in health care protection means creating more constraints on the demand for medical care, especially among employees. In general, it can be inferred that people in Wuhan have a somewhat complex or mixed attitude toward the reform of their health care system—but it is not at all one-sided. This complex pattern is not surprising, as in the literature on public opinion on social policy, people elsewhere have also exhibited a stronger identification with symbolic political beliefs and ideologies about public services that are remote from them but are critical when the issue affects their financial well-being and interest.[21]

Conclusion

The findings of the two social surveys in Wuhan conducted at the end of 2003 are closely examined in this chapter to see whether and how far health care reform has the support of its principal stakeholders. On the basis of these findings, it is fair to suggest that most of the respondents are, in principle, supportive of health care reform (table 5.10, statements 1 and 2). They also basically endorse the three main components of health care reform—the Basic Health Insurance scheme in particular (table 5.4, statements 1, 2, and 3)—and are generally in favor of the reform of medical establishments (we confined ourselves to the study of the effects of reform initiatives on hospitals, table 5.5, statements 1–5) but have mixed feelings about the reform of medicine production and circulation system (here, we confined ourselves to the study of the control of the cost of medicines, table 5.6, statements 1–4).

Larger than the content of these components are the underlying policy and ideological shifts—whether the stakeholders' perceptions of health care reform in Wuhan indicate an endorsement of the policy and ideological shifts. The evidence seems not to be crystal clear. Most of the respondents exhibited a firm support of welfarism, implying that they still preferred the old ethos that the state is primarily responsible for basic health care protection (table 5.7, statements 1, 2, 5, and 6). But, at the same time, many of them also accepted the reciprocal exchange between fees and health care protection, in the case of medical insurance (table 5.7, statement 4). However, they were sensible enough to endorse out-of-pocket payments for health care beyond basic levels (table 5.8, statements 1–4). They also found that medical expenses had already exceeded the affordable levels of the economy and of the general public (table 5.9, statements 2 and 3). More specifically, they worried about the heavy individual responsibility for medical expenses, not only in the present but also in the future, in relation to their own retirement (table 5.10, statements 3–7).

On the basis of this discussion, it is fair to conclude that initiatives of health care reform, in the case of their implementation in Wuhan, a mid-China city, had the general support of two major stakeholders. However, the overall objective of providing better-quality medical services at affordable prices to the common people was still an ideal. But more important are the endorsement of the policy and ideological underpinnings of health care reform. First, people in Wuhan accepted individual responsibility for health care protection; this can be interpreted as an indirect endorsement of the policy notion of privatization, implying that there is a commitment for sharing of responsibilities, through market operations such as out-of-pocket payment, in the new health care system. Second, they also regarded the state as having the primary responsibility for health care, and it was indispensable. Third, the policy shift had also been accompanied by a profound shift in the mix of ideologies underpinning health care reform; if welfarism was the prior ideological base, it still holds a center stage but has to share its ground with neo-liberalism, as reflected by the inroad of individual responsibility into the new health care system and the strong ethos of affordable medical services in line with economic standards, in general, and people's wallets, in particular. Evidently on the last ideology, the present scenario is far from ideal.

Clearly, our survey findings provide a cross-sectional examination of health care reform in a mid-China city. It is not methodologically safe to suggest that the attitudes and beliefs exhibited through the findings were simply reflective of health care reform initiatives. There might be some other factors, such as the effect of prior and concurrent social security reform, retirement protection, in particular, and economic reform, in general. Nevertheless, these cross-sectional findings provide the readers with a snapshot on health care reform at a particular point of time in a specific context. They are useful if the time and context factors are clearly specified.

It is also clear that, in this study, the employee group had generally exhibited more dissatisfaction and worries than the patient group. This is indicative of the realities of economic reform, in general, and health care reform, in particular. It is clear that a socialist state is, in principle, an employee or worker's state. Employees, those of the state-owned enterprises in particular, are the privileged class in a socialist state. Now, China has a market-socialist economy, which is also a prescription of the late Patriarch Deng Xiao-ping, who first initiated economic reform in 1978, aiming to rescue China from a sluggish and underdeveloped economy. In this course of economic reform, evidently the benefits of employees needed to be sliced in order to pave the ground for the emergence of an economy that can compete in the global market. Against this economic context, health care benefits of state employees and state-owned enterprise employees are definitely adversely affected. Our comparative analysis of findings between the employee and patient groups toward health care reform confirms this general observation of the effects of the new distributive system in the new economic order in the case of the employees.

Moreover, it is not methodologically safe to generalize the findings to the larger China and beyond the two stakeholders—employees and hospital patients. Given the fact that these two respondent groups are the privileged few and Wuhan is a latecomer in health care reform, especially in the case of the Basic Health Insurance; hence, those who are less privileged and do not have insurance coverage are more likely to be worse off. Heavy medical cost remains a critical issue for policy makers in China, albeit the Chinese people seem to accept their newfound individual responsibility, which was something unknown to them prior to economic reform.

Notes

1. Similar situations are also found elsewhere. For example, in the case of social security, the profound change is assessed more on the policy and ideological shift from the state to the market and other nonstatutory sectors in terms of responsibility. A good discussion of this can be found in Mark Hyde and John Dixon "Welfare Ideology, the Market and Security: Toward a Typology of Market-Oriented Reform," in *The Marketization of Social Security*, ed. Mark Hyde and John Dixon (Westport, CT: Quorum, 2001), 51–80.

2. Wuhan Statistical Bureau, www3.wuhan.gov.cn (accessed 29 April 2004) (in Chinese).

3. Wuhan Statistical Bureau, "Statistical Release of 2003 National Economic and Social Development of Wuhan City," www.whtj.gov.cn/tjgb/2003NGB.htm (accessed 23 February 2004) (in Chinese).

4. *Ibid.*

5. *Ibid.*

6. Wuhan City Mayor's 2004 working report to the Wuhan City People Representative Congress on 9th January 2004. (in Chinese)

7. Wuhan Statistical Bureau, "Statistical Release."

8. *Ibid.*, see also Wuhan Statistical Bureau, "*Wuhan Statistical Yearbook*, 2003," www.whtj.gov.cn/whtjnj/tjnj2003/2y/index.htm (accessed 23 April 2004) (in Chinese).

9. *Ibid.*

10. Colleen M. Flood, *International Health Care Reform: A Legal, Economic and Political Analysis* (London & New York: Routledge, 2000).

11. Ritu Wu, "Establishing and Perfecting a System of Multi-Layered Medical Insurance." *China Labor* 163 (June 1999):11.

12. Ministry of Health, "*Summary of China's Health Statistics 2004*," www.moh.gov.cn/statistics. *See* also Table 6.6 in chapter 6. (in Chinese)

13. Zi-you Yu, et al., "Health Care Expenses and Reform in China," *WCCS Papers* 7. no. 2 (March 1997): 3.

14. One source is the finding of our field visit to Shenzhen's Labor and Social Security Bureau on 19 November 2003.

15. For examples, Ramon A. Castano, et al., "Equitable Financing, Out-of-Pocket Payments and the Role of Health Care Reform in Colombia," *Health Policy and Planning* 17, no. 1 (2002): S5–S11; Jun Gao, et al., "Health Equity in Transition from Planned to Market Economy in China," *Health Policy and Planning* 17, no. 1 (2002): S20–S29; Wynand P. M. M. van de Ven, "Equity, Cost Containment and Efficiency in Health Care: Can They Be Achieved by Regulated Competition?" in *Ageing, Social Security and Affordability*, ed. T.R. Marmor and P.R. De Jong (Brookfield, VT: Ashgate, 1998).

16. Dong-jin Wang, "The Importance and Urgency of Sufficiently Understanding the Reform of Medical Insurance System for Urban Staff and Workers," *China Labor* (January 1999): 4 (in Chinese); Chack-kie Wong, "Reforming China's State Socialist Workfare System: A Cautionary and Incremental Approach," *Issues and Studies* 35, no. 5 (September/October 1999): 169–194.

17. James Midgley and Kwong-leung Tang, "Social Policy, Economic Growth and Developmental Welfare," *International Journal of Social Welfare* 10, no. 4 (2001): 244–252; Kwong-leung Tang and Raymond Ngan, "China: Developmentalism and Social Security." *International Journal of Social Welfare* 10, no. 4 (2001): 253–259.

18. Chack-kie Wong and Nan-shong P. Li, "Popular Belief in State Intervention for Social Protection in China," *Journal of Social Policy* 29, no. 1 (2000): 109–116.

19. *Ibid.* Wong, (1999).

20. *See* Joe C.B. Leung and Richard. C. Nann, *Authority and Benevolence, Social Welfare in China* (Hong Kong: The Chinese University Press, 1995).

21. Paul Allen Beck, Hal G. Rainery and Carol Traut, "Disadvantage, Disaffection, and Race as Divergent Bases for Citizen Fiscal Policy Preferences," *Journal of Politics* 52, no. 1 (February 1990): 71–93; Olli E. Kangas, "Self Interest and the Common Good: the Impact of Norms, Selfishness and Context in Social Policy Opinions," *Journal of Socio-Economics* 26. no. 5 (1997): 475–494.

Chapter 6

Impact of Health Care Reform

Introduction

The central question in this chapter is whether health care reform, and the full implementation of basic medical insurance, in particular, has advanced in terms of equity. In the preceding chapter, the subjective perceptions of two key stakeholders of the health care system in the case of Wuhan, a mid-China city, were presented. The findings of the two social surveys provide us with a cross-sectional snapshot at a moment when health care reform had moved from its experimental stage to full national implementation, signified by the promulgation of the 1998 Decree on the Decision concerning the Establishment of a Medical Insurance System for Urban Staff and Workers. As mentioned earlier, the national implementation of health care reform is centered on three major components—the introduction of a medical insurance program covering the basic medical needs of urban workers, the reform of medical establishments, and the reform of the medicine production and circulation system. Between 1998 and 2000, the relevant authorities had worked out, step-by-step, a comprehensive reform package covering these three reform initiatives. In this chapter, we present the qualitative data from three focus group interviews, looking for clues on the initial impact of health care reform from the perspective of stakeholders.

Focus group interviews are used to supplement the cross-sectional survey findings with discursive material providing insights into how those who are affected see the new reality of health care reform, especially in terms of equity. The findings from the group interviews are used to identify the initial impact of the new health care system, which has been in place for only a few years. We then ask the basic question, on the basis of a comparative analysis, of whether the new health care system has achieved what it was designed to achieve, the provision of quality health care at affordable costs to average people, and whether it is an equitable and sustainable health care system.

A Brief Preview of Equity in Health Care

Equity has always been a critical issue to China's health care system.[1] Access to health care has primarily been based on employment—employment status, performance, and ownership of the employer[2]—and the place of residence, that is, the divide between rural and urban residence according to household registration.[3] This employment dividing line was institutionalized through the provisions of Government Insurance System, the publicly funded health system for government and public agency employees, and the Labor Insurance System for state-owned enterprise employees in China's urban setting. Both insurance systems were designed for urban employees and were exclusive in coverage. The newly introduced Basic Health Insurance continues this fundamental feature but with two important changes—the transfer of management of medical expenses from individual employers to collective management by social insurance centers, and the extension of insurance cover to employees of all other ownership types.

Despite these changes, the Chinese urban health care system is still characterized by the exclusion and underprotection of those who are uninsured and underinsured.[4] For example, a report identifies five vulnerable groups in 2002 in Shanxi Province (山西省), totalling two million workers or ex-workers of varying status, and a further 580,000 poor, most of them in old age and chronically ill, who were covered by the official poverty relief scheme, the livelihood guarantee allowance,[5] but who had health access problems under the new health care system. The five groups were: (1) 121,000 employees of unprofitable enterprises; (2) 452,000 unemployed and *xiagang* workers; (3) 832,000 retired workers on low pension benefits; (4) 257,000 handicapped; and (5) 240,000 migrant workers.[6] Apparently, all five groups were likely victims in terms of health care access because of their weak employment status in an open economy. It is worth noting that Shanxi Province had more urban poor in China at that time.[7] But the problem of access to health care is not confined to Shanxi Province; it is a nation-wide problem. Even in Beijing, China's capital, a similar situation is reported. A survey conducted in 2001 by the Ministry of Civil Affairs (民政部), the government department responsible for poverty relief and social welfare for the poor and vulnerable groups, and the People's University of China on the vulnerable groups in health care protection in Beijing revealed that three quarters of the respondents chose self-medication to treat their illnesses; the same size of respondents relied on self-payment to finance their medical expenses; only about one-tenth of respondents had Government Insurance and only 2.2 percent had Labor Insurance.[8]

These findings should not be surprising because health care reform does not moderate the basic feature of China's urban health care system—its defining base remains tied to employment. Even worse, economic reform has also brought about widening income gaps. A social scientist at the China

Academy of Social Science estimated that the Gini Coefficient was 0.45 when China first reached the per capita GDP threshold of US$1,000 in 2003,[9] while the vulnerable groups (those mentioned in the previous situtation) are likely to be underinsured or uninsured. This is not to suggest that health care reform does not mitigate inequity in health care at all. The pilot experiment in Zhenjiang is a case in point. A study using data from the annual surveys of the pilot experiment between 1994 and 1996 revealed that the new medical insurance led to a significant increase in outpatient consultations by lower socioeconomic groups and more equitable care for people with chronic illnesses regardless of individual characteristics, but lower socioeconomic groups continued to be disadvantaged in their access to expensive and advanced diagnostic technologies.[10]The study concluded that the pilot urban medical insurance contributed to greater horizontal equity in terms of access to basic health care in some respects but that vertical equity remained constant.

Following this brief preview, we now turn to examine whether the recent full implementation of urban health care reform has had any obvious impact in terms of equitable access to health care, especially for the vulnerable groups. We first present the findings of the focus group interviews.

Findings of the Focus Group Interviews

Three groups of stakeholders in Wuhan were selected for focus group interviews in January 2004, subsequent to the two social surveys. The first group consisted of seven insured people from the same workplace; the second consisted of five officials from Wuhan's social insurance center; and the third consisted of six personnel from two medical establishments—a Chinese medical hospital and a health clinic. The respondents were not meant to be representative in terms of their respective backgrounds. The primary objective of the focus group interviews was to provide supplementary firsthand data, of a discursive kind, in addition to quantitative survey data, to facilitate a deeper understanding of health care reform as it progresses in this mid-China city. It is hoped that focus group interview data will provide a supplementary dataset that will enhance our understanding of health care reform in China.

In this section, the discursive interview findings of the three stakeholder groups are reported in the following order—first, the insured employees; second, the medical insurance center officials; and third, the medical personnel.

The Insured Employees in the Workplace

The workplace for the insured employees was a state-owned enterprise in the manufacturing sector that produces wireless electrical products. There were six employees, three male workers and three female workers; they included an officer-in-charge and a party secretary. All were middle-aged, from thirty-five to fifty-four. According to the respondents, the enterprise was not profitable, but a year and a half earlier it had been publicized as a model enterprise for its early participation in the Basic Health Insurance scheme in Wuhan. It seems that the interviewed employees as a group were not satisfied with the new medical insurance arrangements. Affordability was perceived as the primary concern for them. A few quotes are cited here to illustrate their major worries:

> If I have spent all the money in my (personal saving) account, I need to pay out of my own pocket. Therefore, nowadays, treatment for minor and chronic illnesses will be delayed until (I have) a serious illness. (Male, 46, officer-in-charge)

> Today was my first visit to a hospital . . . over the past one and half years. I have already been coughing for a few months. One of my sisters has cancer, and I feel afraid and have sought medical consultation. After medical consultation in the hospital, I went to a drugstore to buy medicine because it was less expensive. Now I am very worried about what can be done if I have a serious illness. (Male, 35, party cadre)

> I don't know my physical condition. . . . I don't want to have body check because I have no money. If I find out something undesirable and I have no money to pay, I will be very worried and will die earlier. It is better to be folly. (Male, 54, driver)

Clearly, delayed treatment is a common coping method due to insufficient savings in the respondents' personal medical accounts. The first phase in the Three-Phase Passage Model is designed to eliminate abuse in the form of unnecessary reliance on the health services. However, the requirement to use personal medical accounts to pay for medical consultations and drugs has the undesired additional effect of suppressing the treatment of genuine medical needs as well.

Similarly, the new arrangements for medical insurance are perceived by the members of the insured group as affecting the behavior of both patients and hospital personnel alike. For instance, two of them expressed concerns about the limited choice of hospitals:

> In principle, the hospital I am supposed to go to depends on the nature of my illness. But now in Wuhan, medical insurance reform sets limits on the choice of hospitals—we cannot patronize the best hospital because it is not on the list. Listed hospitals are usually those with poor conditions and with low standards. (Male, 46, officer-in-charge)

> In cases of acute illness, any hospital should be good enough. However, if it

> is not a listed hospital, reimbursement is not permitted. Therefore, there is no protection for acute illness. (Female, 46, office worker)

Some members felt that hospitals and doctors had better attitudes toward prescriptions following the introduction of the medical insurance scheme:

> Nowadays, doctors have better attitudes. Patients have more choices. The hospital I went to had more control over doctors—they did not over prescribe medicine. (Female, 47, office worker)

> But this does not tackle the fundamental question—they (doctors) do not prescribe quality medicine. Quality medicine is not on the list for reimbursement. (Male, 46, officer-in-charge)

It is overwhelmingly evident that the first group are, so far, not favorably disposed toward health care reform in terms of affordability and accessibility for medical treatments—it suppresses patients' medical needs and sets constraints on their choice of hospitals and drugs. Apparently, affordability for health care is a major issue for the respondent group. The question was then raised whether the changes of health care treatments, as perceived by the respondent group, evoked a sense of inequity on their part. Different clues were provided:

> Workers experience a lot of pain; they have made tremendous contributions but are not rewarded. Government needs to think more about workers. . . . Medical insurance was established, but it is not useful to workers; their situations are worse off day by day. (Female, 47, office worker)

Apparently, unequal treatment of the employees is understood by comparison with the past when employees were well protected. Another respondent measured the state's current financial contribution to Basic Health Insurance against his ideal of fair shares among the concerned parties:

> Enterprises contribute a little bit more; the state also contributes another bit, and individuals also a little bit. Unlike the present arrangements, the state does not contribute a penny; it only collects money from the workers. (Male, 46, officer-in-charge)

The state is perceived as not playing its part in the financing of medical insurance, and this is felt not to be fair. Another respondent also referred to those government activities that are not related to health care but are regarded by him as a waste of public money:

> Image projects like building squares should be cut back. The state should give more money to medical insurance, at least a part of it. The state should not only ask the workers to contribute. . . . The whole country should care more about workers; it should have a preferential policy toward workers. (Male, 35, party cadre chief)

In the perspective of these respondents, the state does not care about workers. The lack of financial contributions from the government is regarded as the core issue. Although the words "inequity" and "unfairness" were not explicitly used during the focus group interview, there was clearly a great sense of injustice among them in connection with the medical benefits they were entitled to and the part played by the state in the new medical insurance arrangements. The insured workers had the feeling that they were worse off in the new medical insurance scheme. The state is, in their thinking, at least partly responsible for their insufficient health care protection. The medical insurance scheme sets unreasonable constraints on their use of medical services, and insufficient financial input from the government is perceived as a major factor contributing to this.

The Officials at the Medical Insurance Center

The medical insurance center is under the direct administration of Wuhan's Labor and Social Security Bureau. Five officials, three male and two female, from three units of the center—finance, business, and information—were invited to attend the second focus group interview. They were young, aged twenty-five to twenty-eight, which is not surprising given that this is a new social-security-administration organ. In general, the respondents expressed a positive view, favorable to the official line, on the impact of health care reform. It was stressed that medical insurance is important to the economic development and social stability of Wuhan. One suggested that

> The medical insurance system protects the physical health of individual workers by providing proper medication. In this regard, it guarantees the sustainability of human resources for enterprise, government, and public agencies. With this protection, it also guarantees economic development of the district and fosters social stability of the larger society. (Male, 28, Information unit)

On the other hand, the same official did not deny the difficulties and complications of the new system.

> First, complication in types of personnel; complication in age; diversity in occupations; it is easy to have problems. Second, whether enterprises are profitable also affects workers' continued payment for insurance. Some enterprises pay only a month's insurance fee, and they cannot afford any more. However, the workers may not understand and think that the insurance suspension is the fault of the government and have a lot of unreasonable complaints. (Male, 28, Information unit)

On the question of high insurance fees, another official responded that

> It is because previously employees of government and public agencies were entitled to the benefits of the Government Insurance System, therefore there

> are a lot of complaints. Medical insurance has adversely affected the interest of some people from these units. But, medical insurance is welcome by enterprises and the society. (Male, 27, Finance unit)

In response to the question of whether medical insurance guarantees people's needs for medical care, the officials were quite positive. According to one official, the system, even in the short time since its implementation, has already demonstrated its tremendous effects for low-income people.

> It was particularly bad in the past for those families with difficulties. They were not able to benefit from medical protection due to their enterprises' loss-making or some other reasons; medical expenses were a burden to them. Nowadays, medical insurance has already been implemented; their demands for medical care are basically met. (Male, 25, Business unit)

Another cited the small share of fees paid by individual insurers in the case of serious illness, claiming that the new system puts less burden on people—employees and retirees need pay only 20 percent and 15 percent, respectively, of medical expenses, while the socially pooled fund shoulders the rest. She concluded that

> Seemingly, the share paid by individuals is relatively small. Seriously ill patients should be able to foot the bill. (Female, 26, Finance unit)

Another admitted that there is inadequate protection for chronically ill patients, and that the conditions surrounding the authorized lists of drugs, access to medical examinations, and choice of hospitals are stringent. But he defended the system, saying that

> Our medical insurance system is to meet the basic demands of patients in cities. It is not a luxury service. (Male, 27, Finance unit)

Despite the official and positive tone of the views expressed, some inadequacies of the new medical insurance scheme were also mentioned.

The Medical Personnel in Medical Establishments

Six personnel from two medical establishments—one being a Chinese medical hospital, the other a health clinic—were invited for the last focus group interview. Four of them were doctors; the remaining two were hospital administrators. All of them but one were male and were aged from twenty-seven to thirty-six.

To the question of whether the average people in Wuhan were able to afford medical care under the new system, this group of medical personnel respondents did not give us a definite answer. They said that it was contingent on many different conditions.

> Minor illnesses can be self-cared. Serious illnesses need an accumulation of funding [in personal medical accounts] and the help of the family. Therefore, it [medical care] is basically affordable. (Male, 27, hospital medical insurance business unit person-in-charge)

> They [seriously and chronically ill patients] do not need to pay much. Nevertheless, medical expenses for serious illness are still difficult for some people. Therefore, it depends on your income and on the kind of illness you have. (Male, 30, health clinic doctor)

> The cost of giving birth to a baby is still high. Therefore, there is the phenomenon of abandoning newborn babies due to the lack of means. (Male, 33, health clinic doctor)

> Xiagang workers have difficulties even for their basic living. They are unable to pay the insurance fee for medical care protection. (Male, 27, hospital medical insurance business unit person-in-charge)

In general, it seems that serious and chronic illnesses still present a problem to people in vulnerable groups in society, especially those who do not have adequate family support, low-income groups, those with little in the way of personal savings and an insufficient balance in their personal medical accounts, those with illnesses that are not insured or fully insured, for example, AIDS and some types of mental illness. Non-working family members are not included in the new medical insurance; they have to take commercial insurance for health care protection. To low-income households, affordability of medical care is still a critical issue. *Xiagang* workers are another group who have major concerns in terms of health care protection. Apparently, horizontal and vertical inequities remain critical issues despite some advancement, in the perspective of the medical personnel.

The interviewed medical personnel also talked about the medical needs of migrant workers. Two explained the reason of their exclusion from medical insurance coverage:

> These people have high mobility; they do not have any definite employment unit. The government does not have any control over them; it is difficult to manage them. (Male, 36, hospital surgeon)

> Nowadays, we do not have a better approach to respond to this question. But we believe that as the income levels of our residents increase, the problem will be solved. (Male, 27, hospital medical insurance business unit person-in-charge)

Inevitably, the critical issue of equity was raised. Some groups are excluded; some medical needs are not covered under the conditions of the new system. However, in one doctor's view, medical insurance is able to meet the basic medical needs of the poor. He used metaphors to illustrate.

> People in poor conditions take congee; better-off people eat meat. You should not prohibit the rich from eating meat, but they have to pay for it from their own pocket. (Male, 30, health clinic doctor)

In other words, medical insurance is about the provision of a basic standard of medical care; a developmental perspective underpins it. This perspective is used to justify the imposition of control over patients' medical care, where their needs go beyond the basic medical standards that China's economic level, and that of Wuhan, can sustain. A hospital administrator described the ways in which the use of drugs is controlled.

> We have medicines for basic use and medicines for non-basic use. In the case of medicines for basic use, doctors must select from the list; in the case of medicines for non-basic use, doctors have to explain the position clearly to patients. (Male, 27, hospital medical insurance business unit person-in-charge)

In a word, patients have to shoulder the costs of non-basic drugs. The "ability to pay" defines the choice of drugs, not the required quality.

We here discuss briefly the control of drugs by the new medical insurance. In accordance with an official document of the Ministry of Labor and Social Security,[11] the drug lists include a combination of Western and Chinese ready-to-use drugs; they are divided into Catalogs A and B. Drugs in Catalog A are clinically essential, widely used, with good clinical effects, and cheap compared with other drugs of the same kind. Catalog A is a nation-wide drug list; local authorities are not allowed to make any changes. Catalog B drugs are more expensive, with the same clinical effects, and are also decided by the relevant authorities of the central government. Nevertheless, local authorities are allowed to amend the list according to local variations in drug-use practice, economic levels, and individual patients' medical needs. However, the total changes for drug items on the local list should not vary by more than 15 percent above or below the total drug items in the catalog.

Indeed, lower-income patients as well as being restricted in their choices of drugs for medication also have to pay medical fees for goods and services that are usually considered essential parts of their medical and hospital care. They have to pay registration fees; they have to pay for the material costs of medical records, costs of ambulance use, and costs of their living expenses during hospitalization, e.g., food.[12]Basic Health Insurance means "basic" in a literal sense. It is reasonable to argue that the vulnerable groups in society are in a more difficult position than their fellow residents in terms of accessibility and affordability of health care.

Hospital administrators and doctors also feel the effects of control. One put it directly in terms of financial implications to hospitals.

> Originally profits from selling drugs were enormous; now they are relatively small but still a large amount. (Male, 33, health clinic doctor)

Moreover, hospitals face financial risks in admitting insured patients. In accordance with the hospital rules, hospitals receive a fixed sum for healing a patient; however, they do not receive the whole of the fixed sum until the end of the year. If a patient does not leave the hospital at the end of the year, the hospital would not be reimbursed until the following year and would have a cash flow problem. In the case of patients who die despite treatment, hospitals might not receive any sum from the patients' families. This is less likely with uninsured patients because they are required to pay most of the medical expenses before treatment.

Apparently, the new medical insurance, unlike the Government Insurance System, which was easily abused by patients and hospitals alike, is harsh toward hospitals in terms of cost control. Nevertheless, hospitals are still able to pass part of the costs to patients. One talked about fee standardization.

> Our hospital charges a standard 15.8 yuan per day to a patient for the use of a bed; however, Basic Health Insurance reimburses us only 9.8 yuan, and the difference has to be borne by patients. (Male, 27, hospital medical insurance business unit person-in-charge)

The stringent reimbursement standard is meant to eliminate abuse by hospitals, but it also hurts patients. Nevertheless, on the basis of the interview findings, there has been much less abuse on the part of hospitals since Basic Health Insurance was put in place.

As mentioned before, the medical personnel seem to be positive toward the new medical insurance. Moreover, they are also optimistic about its future development for the benefit of patients. In the words of a hospital administrator, as more enterprises join the new medical insurance scheme, patients will have more benefits. For example, threshold charges and co-payments will decrease, and more serious illnesses will be included.

> Originally, a ceiling was set for cancer patients, who tended to use all of their money quickly. Now, there is no ceiling for cancer and kidney patients; diabetic and third-stage high blood pressure patients were given more than 5,000 (yuan) last year; later it was changed to 6,494 (yuan). (Male, 27, hospital medical insurance business unit person-in-charge)

In other words, they see a bright future for the insured despite all the present drawbacks. An incremental perspective underpins this optimism. In sum, the three focus group interview findings provide us with insights into how the major stakeholders of the health care system in a mid-China city reacted to the new initiatives in health care reform.

The responses of the insured group are similar to the responses we received in the survey of patients and employees. They reflect dissatisfaction with the suppression of medical needs by the deliberate control of the choice of hospitals, the choice of drug use, and the use of co-payment. Apparently, some have been discouraged by these control arrangements and either delay medical treatment or do not seek it at all, even when they need it. As reflected in these discursive findings, accessibility and affordability of medical care are critical issues for the insured group. They are workers in a socialist state, but they feel that the state does not contribute its fair share in the financing of medical insurance for their benefit. In other words, from the perspective of the insured urban workers, it is reasonable to suggest that the new health care system has not enhanced equity, either vertical or horizontal, and that they are worse off than before. They feel that they have been abandoned by the state.

The officials of the medical insurance center take a different view. They have stuck to the official line by suggesting that the introduction of medical insurance has had a positive impact on economic development and social stability. The primary objective of medical insurance is to provide health care protection at a basic level. At this level, the needs for medical care of the average people, even those families in difficulty, are basically met. In their view, horizontal equity and, to a limited extent, vertical equity have been enhanced.

The medical personnel generally support these official views, especially in regard to the affordability of medical care at a basic level. They suggest that co-payments are fairly low. However, they also admitted frankly that the medical needs of some uninsured groups such as children, migrant workers, and *xiagang* workers are being neglected. However, an optimistic future is projected in view of the incremental move toward enlarged insurance coverage.

The focus group interview findings reveal the subjective responses and judgments of those who hold different positions in China's health care system. It can be argued that the introduction of the three major health care reform components suppress the medical needs of the insured, reduce abuses of hospitals and doctors, and meet the *basic* health care needs of *insured* urban workers at affordable costs. Nevertheless, the term "basic," a discursive concept, is subject to different interpretations—the insured might regard "quality" or "non-basic" drugs as "basic" while the officials and medical personnel take a different view. How can we reconcile these contrary views taken by the three stakeholder groups, the insured on one side and the other two groups on the other, in terms of equity? For a fair assessment, it is necessary, using available statistical data, to place these subjective views in the wider context of China's health care reform. In the following section, China's health care reform is examined in reference to equitable access to health care.

China's Health Care Reform in Proper Perspective

Here, we examine the initial impact of health care reform, which has been in full implementation since 1998, in a wider context. A few earlier studies assessed the pilot project in Zhenjiang in 1994 and found that the experimental insurance plan was effective in containing total health care expenditure.[13] With the full implementation of health care reform in 1998, a similar approach to that of the Zhenjiang pilot experimental model was adopted. Hence, it is reasonable to assume that the full national implementation is likely to have a similar effect in preventing health care costs from escalating unreasonably. For example, according to a Ministry of Health report, outpatient fees rose by 9 percent in 2001; that figure was similar to the 8 percent rise of per capita urban household income in the same year. However, in earlier periods, for example, 1991–1995, the costs of the same medical treatment rose by an annual 26 percent. This rise slowed down to 15 percent in the period between 1996–2000.[14] These calculations did not take the change in consumer price index (CPI) into consideration. In the latter period, China had a much lower CPI.

Even if health care reform is effective in containing monetary costs, questions still need to be asked about other, nonmonetary costs. As was mentioned earlier in our focus group interview with the insured, the medical needs of the insured are suppressed deliberately. Moreover, the officials and medical personnel frankly admitted that vulnerable groups were not covered in the new scheme. Equity remains a critical issue for policy makers. We will begin, however, with what has been achieved in the health care reform. We will then extend the discussion to a wider context in terms of equity, the role of the state, and the financing of health care.

Table 6.1 presents some major figures on the development of basic medical insurance in China in the period between 1998–2003. Taking the financial side first, we notice that basic medical insurance was financially sustainable in this period. The accumulated surplus stood at 980 million yuan in 1998 when 5,093 thousand employees and retirees were insured under the scheme, and by 2003, when the total insured employees and retirees passed the 100 million mark, it had risen to a surplus of 37,900 million. In the year 2000, the numbers of insured suddenly shot up by 629.4 percent from the previous year, to a figure of 43,320 thousand insured employees and retirees. This jump coincided with the full implementation of health care reform between 1998–2000. Turning now to the extent of the coverage—according to a Ministry of Health announcement, nearly all urban areas had established basic medical insurance in 2002. In spite of this, not all urban employees and retirees were participating in the new health insurance scheme. When the total insured passed the 100 million mark, the figures were exactly 109,028 thousand for both employees and retirees, and 79,750 thousand for employees, but these made up only 20.8 percent of the total urban population and only 31 percent of the total urban working population, respectively.[15] In other words, in spite of the success of the scheme in terms of cost containment and the extension of the coverage, the medical needs of the overwhelming majority of urban dwellers were not covered.

This does not mean the introduction of Basic Health Insurance and the accompanying reform initiatives were not helpful in some respects. Table 6.2

Table 6.1 Developments of the Basic Health Insurance in China, 1998–2003

	1998	1999	2000	2001	2002	2003
Employees (in thousands)	4,017	4,698	43,320	54,710	69,260	79,750
Retirees (in thousands)	1,076	1,241		18,150	24,740	29,270
Total (in thousands) (Annual change)	5,093 (Employee:+36% Retirees:+45.7%)	5,939 (+16.6%)	43,320 (+629.4%)	72,8601 (+68.2%)	94,000 (+29.0%)	109,028 (+16.0%)
Cities/Districts	40+	59	284	339	Nearly all	Nearly all
Income (100 million yuan)	19.5	24.5	170	384	607.8	890
Expenditure (100 million yuan)	15.6	16.5	124	244	409.4	654
Accumulated surplus (Deficit) (100 million yuan)	9.8	8	89	253	450.7	379

Source: *Annual Statistical Announcement of the Development of Labor and Social Insurance*, Ministry of Labor and Social Security, PRC. (1998–2003) (In Chinese) www.molss.gov.cn/ (accessed 31 August 2004) (in Chinese)
Note: All are year-end figures.

presents the income and expenditure of general hospitals in China in selected years; it is helpful for us to look at key indicators in their budgets to see whether medical costs were held within budgeted limits and whether they met the objectives of the health care reform in the years between 1998, the beginning of full implementation, and 2000, when there was a very substantial rise in the numbers insured (see table 6.1).

The figures in table 6.2 suggest that general hospitals in China relied heavily on their business income from patient care, both outpatient and inpatient, between 1990–2001, and their medical and drug income between 2002 and 2003. Government subsidies, both business subsidies and special program subsidies, were minimal and declining over the years since 1990, when they were 9.7 percent and 4.7 percent, respectively, of the business income of the average hospital. Business subsidies and special program subsidies fell to 4.9 percent and 1.9 percent, respectively, in 1998, and then somewhat increased to 5.9 percent and 1.7 percent, respectively, in 1999; they then fell a little to 5.4 percent and 1.5 percent, respectively, in 2000; the respective figures in 2001 were 6.1 percent and 1.8 percent. Despite the change in categorization between 2002 and 2003, when government subsidies were included in medical income, it is reasonable to assume that there would not be much variation in government subsidies—and they remained

Table 6.2 Incomes and expenditures of general hospitals in China, selected years

	1990	1995	1998	1999	2000	2001	2002	2003
No. of hospitals	2,438	3,728	4,052	4,072	4,088	4,112	4,488	4,800
Business income per hospital (10 000 yuan)	484.7	1559.8	2301.7	2576.3	2941.4	3,192.5	3392.9	3661.7
Outpatient (%)	38.8	36.2	40.8	42.1	42.6	42.0		
Inpatient (%)	52.4	53.1	54.3	56.6	56.5	57.2		
Medical income (%)							49.6	49.9
Drug income (%)							47.6	47.3
Business subsidies (%)*	9.7	6.5	4.9	5.9	5.4	6.1		
Special program Subsidies (%)*	4.7	2.6	1.9	1.7	1.5	1.8		
Others (%)							2.7	2.7
Average medical expense per outpatient (yuan)	10.9	39.9	68.8	79.0	85.8	93.6	99.6	108.2
Drug (%)	67.9	64.2	62.1	60.0	58.6	57.7	55.4	54.7
Average medical expense per inpatient (yuan)	473.3	1668.0	2596.8	2891.1	3083.7	3245.5	3597.7	3910.7
Drug (%)	55.1	52.8	49.2	47.2	46.1	45.5	44.4	44.7
Examination and treatment (%)	22.0	25.5	28.1	29.7	31.7	31.6	27.9	26.9

Source: Ministry of Health, PRC *Statistical Summaries of China's Health*, various years. www.moh.gov.cn/tjxxzx/tjsj/tjty/index.htm (accessed 31 August 2004) (in Chinese)
*These two percentages illustrate their share of the business income per hospital, as the total income per hospital is not provided in the original tables.

a minimal part of the total income of an average general hospital in China. In contrast, in 2003, in Hong Kong—a special administrative region in China, which like Macau has a different economic system from the rest of China—the Hospital Authority, which manages all public hospitals, had 92.8 percent of its income from public revenue while fees and charges consisted of 2.7 percent.[16]

Apparently, since the early 1980s, the inadequate funding from the government has forced hospitals to rely upon other sources for revenue, as we mentioned earlier.[17] Drug and medical examinations were two key revenue generators. This was especially the case with sales of drugs, which, it has been suggested, is the underlying structural factor for the "runaway" increases in medical costs. The use of drug sales as the main income was coined "*yiyao yangyi*".[18] In this sense, the cost of drugs to patients should be a good and reliable indicator of whether the health care reforms have been fully implemented, given that one of the aims of the reform is to achieve reductions in the costs of drugs in each medical consultation.

In 1990, 67.9 percent of the average medical cost per outpatient in general hospital treatment was for drugs. The ratio fell to 62.1 percent in 1998. It fell further to 54.7 percent in 2003 (see table 6.2). The continuing falls in the share of drug costs in outpatient medical expenses happened prior to the full nationwide implementation of the health care reform initiatives between 1998 and 2000. If the jump in the numbers of insured in 2000 is taken as the transition point, this means that the transfer from Government Insurance and Labor Insurance to the new medical insurance should be followed by a corresponding fall in the share of drug costs in outpatient medical expenses in 2000, and more especially in 2001, when the full impact of the 629.4 percent rise in the number of insured was felt.

However, the fall in drug costs as a percentage of the average medical cost per outpatient proceeded at the same slow rate in 2002 and 2003. The same pattern is also seen in relation to inpatient treatments (see table 6.2). Apparently, the spread of the reform did not bring about any obvious clear-cut change in the average medical expenses of either outpatient treatment or inpatient treatment in general hospitals in China. It seems that the fall in the ratio of drug expenses as a share of total medical treatment in China's general hospitals was normalized before health care reform was fully implemented. In this regard, it is necessary to look for further indicators to see whether health care reform has had any positive effects on total health expenditure. We shall come back to this issue later in this chapter.

Table 6.3 looks at the sources of financing for the health care system in China between two points in time. The information comes from two national surveys on health services across China, conducted by the Ministry of Health in 1998 and 2003. They were large-scale national surveys, which covered very large populations. In the second national health survey conducted in 1998, 123,063 households with 469,568 people, of which 87.2 percent were rural residents, were interviewed.[19]The full details of the 2003 third national survey have not yet been disclosed except for the previously mentioned data. The data from 1998 can be used as the reference point, while the changes in 2003 can be seen as an effect of the health care reform initiatives, given that there was no other significant policy change in the period. The data on urban respondents are reported here.

Looking at the distribution of the sources of finance in China's health care system, first, the remarkable thing is that, in 1998, 44.1 percent of the finance came from self-payment, while the figure in 2003 was remained at roughly the same level, i.e., 44.8 percent. Both figures are high. Second, there were significant increases in the financing from social insurance. For example, the share of social insurance in terms of basic insurance and serious illness insurance rose very substantially over the period, from 4.7 percent in 1998 to 32.2 percent in 2003—a 27.5 percentage-point increase over just five years. It can be assumed

Table 6.3 Sources of finance of China's urban health care, 1998 and 2003 (%)

	1998	2003
Social insurance (basic insurance, serious illness insurance)	4.7	32.2
Government Insurance	16.0	4.0
Labor Insurance	28.7	4.6
Cooperative insurance	2.7	6.6
Commercial insurance	/	5.6
Self-payment	44.1	44.8
Other	3.7	2.2
Total	99.9	100.0

Source: Ministry of Health, PRC *National Survey on Health Service* in 1998, 2003, see 2003 and 2004 *China Health Statistics Summary*. Ministry of Health, PRC. www.moh.gov.cn/statistics/digest03/t28.htm (accessed 31 August 2004) (in Chinese)

that the contribution of social insurance to the financing of China's urban health care system will grow further, given the trend that we noticed in the statistics in table 6.1. Other medical insurance programs, such as cooperative insurance for the rural population in the periphery of the cities and commercial insurance primarily for topping up the benefits for the urban insured population, were on the rise—from 2.7 percent in 1998 to 6.6 percent in 2003 in the case of the former, and from zero in 1998 to 5.6 percent in 2003 in the case of the latter.

Third, table 6.3 unveils a significant fall in the state financing of health care. Finance from Government Insurance fell from 16.0 percent in 1998 to 4.0 percent in 2003, while in Labor Insurance state funding was also reduced from 28.7 percent in 1998 to 4.6 percent in 2003. Both medical insurance programs represent the state's health care protection for government, public agency, and state-owned enterprise employees. Apparently, the financing of China's health care system has shifted toward relying on social insurance, with the rapid expansion of basic medical insurance in the period under study.

In sum, it can be inferred that medical insurance of different types, social insurance, and other types as well have had a significant impact on the financing of China's urban health care system in the short period under study, that is, between 1998 and 2003, when the three major components of health care reform were fully implemented. In other words, there has been a systemic shift alongside the reform initiatives. However, the systemic shift in health care financing did not have any impact on the levels of self-payment—out-of-pocket payments from personal funding at the two points of time were both at significantly high levels. Moreover, the role played by the state in health care financing has reduced substantially, in a relative sense; the evidence here is the fall in the shares of Government Insurance and Labor Insurance over this period in China's urban health care system. The share of total government health costs also fell substantially in the same period. We shall refer to the figures in table 6.6. In terms of the sources of finance in China's health care system, the figures do not reflect a pattern of diminishing affordability and accessibility to health care for the average person—out-of-pocket payments remained constant over the period under examination. Out-of-pocket payment is a regressive form of health care finance; it is especially unfair to the poor and the vulnerable groups. Hence, health care reform did not do any particular favors in mitigating the health care burden of the poor and the vulnerable groups in China. Moreover, the Government Insurance System and Labor Insurance System insured employees were worse off because they were transferred to a medical insurance scheme that deliberately suppressed their medical needs. It is also worth noting that, from the perspective of the authorities, the traditional health care system was unable to control unreasonable consumption —the broad range of medical benefits remained at little or no cost to workers.

Given that the full implementation of health care reform did not mitigate the financial burden of those with medical needs, the issue of equity in health care remained critical to the urban population and to vulnerable groups in particular. Apparently, the new urban health care system has institutionalized various constraining measures for suppressing medical needs and for controlling abuses by hospitals and doctors; however, further expansion of social insurance may not be able to reduce out-of-pocket payments by the insured. The impact of health care reform, seemingly, was a shift from the old forms of insurance, i.e., Government Insurance and Labor Insurance, to new forms of insurance, both social and commercial, in which the role of the state is financially minimal. In other words, affordability is still a critical issue for many people, vulnerable groups in particular, despite the state's reform efforts. Thus, equity remains a matter of concern, as those who need medical treatment still do not have access to it.

The Impact of Minimal State Financing

The systemic shift in the sources of finance in China's health care system reflects an institutional arrangement in which there is minimal funding by the state coupled with strong state regulation and enforcement. Table 6.3 vividly illustrates the effective shift in the financing pattern—the full implementation of health care reform did not alter the amounts of self-payment but brought about a substantial shift from government- and employer-financed insurance to joint employer-employee-financed social insurance. The empirical data of the 1998 national health survey is helpful in revealing the social costs of this arrangement in terms of equity.

Since the complete findings of the third National Health Survey were not available, those of the second national survey in 1998 were examined. It is reasonable to assume that the findings five years earlier in the second national survey should be reflective of the third national survey because the share of self-payments as a source of the financing of health care remained the same between these two points in time (see table 6.3). Table 6.4 looks at the underlying reasoning of those who chose self-medication for medical treatment and of those who discharged themselves from hospitals. Of the urban respon-

Table 6.4 Survey findings of the reasons for self-medication and self-requested discharges of urban residents from hospitals in 1998 National Health Survey

Survey items	
Self-medication	
(Number of respondents)	(4,447)
Of the total respondents (%)	43.9
The reason for not taking any medication (%)	
Feeling of minor illness	39.06
Financial difficulties	32.28
Lack of time	3.31
Inconvenience due to transportation	0.16
Too wasteful of time	1.26
Poor attitudes	0.16
Lack of effective treatment	9.45
Other	14.33
Reasons for self-discharging from hospitals (%)	
(Number of respondents)	(2,243)
Got better; on request of doctors	48.33
Did not get better, but on request of doctors	9.09
Self-request discharges	36.47
Other	6.11
Reasons for self-requested discharges from hospitals (%)	
(Number of respondents)	(818)
Cannot get well	13.08
Financial difficulties	45.72
Limited conditions of hospitals	4.65
Poor service attitudes	1.10
Other	35.45

Source: Ministry of Health, PRC. 1998 *National Health Survey Analytical Report*. www.moh.gov.cn/statistics/ronhs98/index.htm (accessed 31 August 2004) (in Chinese)
Note: The respondents were asked about their health conditions and medical treatments in the previous two weeks.

-dents who adopted self-medication for medical treatment, 32.28 percent did so due to financial difficulties. Of those who discharged themselves from hospitals, 36.47 percent did so at their own request; among them, 45.72 percent did so due to financial difficulties.

These findings from the National Health Survey are compatible with our survey findings reported in the previous chapter and those of the focus group interview findings presented in the earlier section in this chapter. Apparently, affordability is a critical issue for a substantial part of the urban population; it is quite reasonable to predict that vulnerable groups such as the poor, *xiagang* workers, and migrant workers are disproportionately and adversely affected. Some of the findings of the social surveys in Wuhan are repeated here for illustration—62.9 percent of both employee and patient respondents agree that "the current individual responsibility for medical expenses is too heavy" (table 5.10, statement 3); and 64.9 percent of both employee and patient respondents agree that "it is common that people are afraid of seeking medical consultation when they are ill in Wuhan" (table 5.10, statement 4).

A cross tabulation of respondents' socioeconomic and demographic backgrounds with the responding pattern reveals that common social vulnerability characteristics are the predictors—elderly, less educated, lower-income, and state-owned enterprise employee respondents felt their individual responsibility for medical expenses as a heavier burden (table 6.5, statement 1), and elderly and lower-income respondents shied away from medical treatment when they were ill in Wuhan (table 6.5, statement 2). All the differences on socioeconomic and demographic backgrounds had statistical significance. Perhaps it is worth outlining the size of those who were likely to be in a socially vulnerable position in Wuhan. According to the official figures, at the end of 2003, 7.5 percent, or 585 thousand people, in Wuhan were aged 65 and older; there were 1.3 million employees of state-owned enterprises; and there were also 3.4 million instances of the provision of the state poverty relief in the same period.[20]

Our discursive interview findings, especially from the insured group, also confirm the findings of the aggregate statistical data of the two social surveys. It is thus reasonable to assume that traditional vulnerable groups in society are likely to have problems in terms of access to medical treatment in the present health care system, despite the recent enforcement of three major reform components in the period between 1998 and 2000. Equity is about fairness; hence, the unfair allocation of perceived individual responsibility for medical costs and the affordability of health care are unequivocally an equity issue.

Here, we turn to the issue of minimal state financing as the underlying force driving the formation of the new urban health care system in China. In this system, hospitals have to maximize their income from drug sales and medical examinations using expensive diagnostic technologies, to keep their budgets in balance. In other words, the minimal financial role of the state was likely an important initiator of the shift toward the new system, along with the problems of inflated costs

Table 6.5 Perceived individual responsibility and affordability cross-tabulated with sociodemographic and economic backgrounds of respondents in Wuhan, 2003 (%)

	Age			Education			Personal Income			Employment Type			Ownership	
	18–30	31–59	60 or older	Primary or below	Secondary	Tertiary or above	Below ¥1000	¥1000–¥1999	¥2000 or above	Permanent	Contracted	Temporary	Stated owned	Other types
1. The current individual responsibility on medical expenses is:														
Too heavy	48.1	66.8	85.0	87.5	70.9	54.9	70.6	68.8	52.2	64.2	58.3	50.0	69.3	54.2
Just fine	47.5	31.0	10.0	12.5	25.7	41.1	26.8	28.9	43.4	34.0	36.7	50.0	28.5	41.0
Can bear more	4.4	2.2	5.0	3.4	4.0	2.6	2.3	4.4	1.9	5.0			2.2	4.7
(N)	(181)	(232)	(80)	(32)	(179)	(275)	(153)	(173)	(113)	(162)	(60)	(4)	(277)	(212)
X_2		39.383***			21.215***			11.467*			2.440		12.275**	
2. It is common that people are afraid of seeking medical advice when they are ill in Wuhan.														
Agree	54.5	69.5	74.7	79.4	65.3	64.2	72.1	68.4	56.0	66.5	66.2	85.7	68.5	60.9
Half-half	28.2	15.0	16.8	14.7	16.3	22.6	15.2	17.1	26.1	20.6	22.1	14.3	17.7	22.9
Disagree	17.2	15.4	8.4	5.9	18.4	13.3	12.7	14.5	17.9	12.9	11.8		13.8	16.3
(N)	(209)	(266)	(95)	(34)	(196)	(332)	(165)	(193)	(134)	(194)	(68)	(7)	(305)	(258)
X_2		19.956**			8.110		9.744*				1.511		3.711	

*$p < 0.05$; ** $p < 0.01$; *** $p < 0.001$

Note: Employment type included only employee respondents.

due to unconstrained consumption on the part of the workers in the traditional health care system. The new health care system is characterized by high out-of-pocket payments, large groups of the population without access to basic health care, and medical costs that are still, both in absolute and relative terms, surprisingly high. Table 6.6 illustrates this scenario.

We start with the "World Health Report 2000" as the backdrop for table 6.6. The World Health Organization report had the following noble aim:

> The report sets out to analyze the role of health systems and suggest how to make them more efficient and, most important, more accessible and responsive to the hundreds of millions of people presently excluded from benefiting fully from them. . . . For all their achievements and good intentions, health systems have failed globally to narrow the health divide between rich and poor in the last 100 years. In fact, the gap is actually widening. Some such worsening often accompanies economic progress, as the already better-off are the first to benefit from it. [21]

Table 6.6 China's health care expenses and national wealth, 1980–2002 (at current prices)

	1980	1990	1995	1997	1998	1999	2000	2001	2002
Total health expenses (100 million yuan)	14.32	743.0	2,257.8	3,384.9	3,776.5	4,178.6	4,764.0	5,150.3	5,684.6
Government health expenses (%)	36.2	25.0	17.0	15.4	15.6	15.3	14.9	15.5	15.2
Social health expenses (%)	42.6	38.0	32.7	27.7	26.6	25.5	24.5	24.0	26.5
Individual health expenses (%)	21.2	37.0	50.3	56.9	57.8	59.2	60.6	60.5	58.3
Per capita health expenses (yuan)	14.51	65.0	190.6	273.8	302.6	5.10	376.4	403.6	442.6
Total health expenses as % of GDP	3.17	4.00	3.86	4.55	4.82	331.9	5.33	5.37+	5.42
GDP (100 million yuan)	451.8	18,548	58,478	74,463	78,345	82,068	89,442	95,933	104,882

Notes:

1. Because of statistical adjustment, total health expenses in 2001 do not include health education at tertiary level and residents' expenses on preventive medicines.

+ It was revised to 5.16 in 2004. Source: Ministry of Health (2004) *Summary of China's Health Statistics*, 2004. www.moh.gov.cn/ (accessed 5 September 2004) (in Chinese)

This quote from the WHO's report is relevant to our analysis. As we mentioned earlier in this chapter, China was once praised for its achievements in enhancing the health of its people, including the rural residents, in the early decades of Communist rule. In other words, the failure elsewhere of health care systems to narrow the health divide was generally not applicable to the Chinese case in the period when China had the old health care system in place. However, that system was criticized for its deteriorating quality of care, inefficiencies, abuses, and waste; most important, it was incompatible with the transition to an open-market economy—the need to facilitate labor mobility and to lower the cost of production for state-owned enterprises. Hence, health care reform was a necessary and essential step in remedying these systemic faults and in making the smooth transition to an open economy.

The claim in the WHO's report that the rich benefited more from the evolving health care system may not be true in China's case. The rich have to pay more for their health care in China under the new system, just like their less-well-off compatriots. In this sense, the rich are not better off, as suggested in the WHO quote. China's new health care system has outperformed its targeted national growth rates (this point will be illustrated later), while average people, including the rich and especially vulnerable groups, have problems in accessing health care. Here we take a close look at the figures in table 6.6 in an attempt at explaining our observation.

In 1980, during the pre-reform era, China spent only 1,432 million yuan (at current prices, as in what follows) on health care, which was equivalent to 3.17 percent of its gross domestic product (GDP). Twenty-two years later in 2002, the health care costs had increased 39.7 times to 568,460 million yuan, 5.42 percent of GDP. GDP did not increase as fast as health care costs, increasing only by a factor of 23.2 times the 1980 figure. It is clear that both in absolute and relative terms, health care costs and health care costs as a percentage of GDP have very substantially increased over a period of more than two decades. Greatly increased resources have been put into China's health care system, but they have produced results that, on the basis of the previous discussion, are less than satisfactory. One possible explanation lies in the shift in the share of costs amongst different sectors—the shift had become increasingly unfavorable to individuals and society.

The continued falls in the share of drug expenses per inpatient and per outpatient as a proportion of the total cost of hospital treatment (see table 6.2) seem less significant in the light of the failure to prevent increases in the overall cost of health care. This failure is evidenced by the growth in total health costs as a percentage of GDP in the two years following 2000, the year in which the full implementation of the health care reform took place.

Evidently, the role of the state in health care funding was much more significant in 1980, at the beginning of China's economic reform, when the government funded 36.2 percent of the total health care costs, and the respective shares from society and individuals were 42.6 and 21.2 percent. The government's share had fallen to 25 percent by 1990. It stabilized over the following twelve years, from 25 percent in 1990, to 17 percent in 1995, to around 15 percent in the years between 1996 and 2002. At the same time, it was also evident that the share of individual payments increased very substantially, from 21.2 percent in 1980 to 37 percent in 1990, to 50.3 percent in 1995, and to the higher end of the fifties between 1997 and 2002. The final figure, in 2002, was 58.3 percent, representing a fall of 2.2 percentage points in one year. It is not yet known whether this was the start of a falling trend, but in any event it is still a very high level of individual payments as a share of total health expenses.

It is fair to conclude that individual out-of-pocket payments as a percentage of total health care expenses in China have become increasingly heavy over the nearly two and a half decades under study. No wonder that the same WHO report ranks China at sixty-one in terms of the level of health of its people, but at 144 in terms of overall health system performance in the 1997 estimates.[22]The former assessment reflects the earlier enormous achievements of China in improving the level of health of its people, which was far beyond what could be expected for China's stage of economic development in the pre-reform era.[23] This can be regarded as evidence that the foundation of China's earlier health achievements—a broad publicly financed and conducted disease prevention strategy and accessible primary health care—was still in place in the reform era.

However, China's achievements in the realm of public health did not spill over to the rest of its health care system, especially in the area of health care finance. Therefore, it is not surprising that its worst rankings in the WHO's reports have been in the area of fairness in financial contributions to the health system—it was ranked 188 (table 6.7) out of the WHO's 191 members states; China outperformed only Brazil, Myanmar, and Sierra Leone. According to the WHO report, fairness in financing health care systems implies that the risks each household faces due to the costs of the health care system are distributed according to ability to pay rather than to the risk of illness, while overall system performance is composed of a measure of achievement in the level of health, the distribution of health, the level of responsiveness, the distribution of responsiveness, and the fairness of financial contribution. In this light, an equitable health care finance system ensures financial protection for everyone. This set of WHO performance indicators positions China's evolving health care system in a proper perspective—it has an equity problem to tackle, not only because of complaints from its own people, as exemplified by the survey findings in Wuhan, but also in comparative terms its system performs poorly in this respect by international standards.

The WHO's league table of health care system performance is a recent innovation, and we therefore do not have earlier benchmarks for a comparison over time. Nevertheless, it would be worthwhile to do a comparative analysis on the basis of the resources put into health care as a percentage of national wealth. Apparently, economic reform has brought enormous wealth to China—its national wealth in terms of GDP has undergone a 23.2 times increase over a period of twenty-two years, 1980–2002 (see table 6.6). It is therefore desirable to assess whether the newly created wealth contributes to an improved,

Table 6.7 China in comparison to countries with comparable levels of GDP spending on health care, 1997

	Health expenditure as % of GDP	On level of health	Overall health system performance	Fairness of financial contribution to health systems
South Korea	5.1	107	58	53
Luxembourg	6.0	31	16	2
Mexico	5.3	63	61	144
Turkey	4.8	33	70	49–50
China	4.6 5.4(2001)	61	144	188

Sources: *World Health Report 2000*; *OECD Health Data 2001.*
Health Ministry, PRC. Source: Ministry of Health (2004) *Summary of China's Health Statistics*, 2004. www.moh.gov.cn/news/sub_index.aspx?tp_class=C3 (accessed 5 September 2004)

well-performing, and more equitable health care system, in terms of cross-national comparisons.

We chose similar levels of health expenditure as a percentage of GDP as the key indicator for comparative analysis. In this light, South Korea, Luxembourg, Mexico, and Turkey are selected for comparison. Table 6.6 illustrates that a similar or slightly higher input of precious national wealth does not produce a similar level of health, overall health system performance, and fairness of financial contribution in the health system. Only in terms of levels of health were two selected countries—South Korea and Mexico—worse than China: 107 for South Korea, 63 for Mexico, and 61 for China (see table 6.7). For the other two indicators, China's respective rankings were far worse than the selected four comparable countries. These selected cross-national comparisons prove an important empirical observation: the health care system matters, regardless of wealth.

Conclusion

Taking our earlier observation that the full implementation of health care reform has not mitigated the financial burden of those who have medical needs, it is now also clear that China's present health care system does not perform well, in comparative terms, despite its being able to draw some comfort from the level of health of its people. Having said that, the evolving health care system still has substantial successes to register, as we outlined in chapter 3. Its co-payment mechanism for employees has reduced the financial burden on employers. On the provider side, doctors are forced to look to the fee guidelines; this has been helpful in containing the rising medical costs. On the quality side, due to the introduction of competition among medical establishments, quality of medical services has improved, and the incidents of unwarranted prescriptions have decreased.

Nevertheless, simply in terms of financial equity and overall system performance, the evolving Chinese health care system is definitely in need of a redirection. The recent urban health care reform could not tackle these issues because, according to our analysis, it did not mitigate the medical expenses of average people, and especially of vulnerable groups. Out-of-pocket payments remained the same subsequent to health care reform.

The transfer of Government Insurance and Labor Insurance to Basic Health Insurance succeeded in reducing the financial role of the state (for instance, from 16 percent in 1998 to 4 percent in 2003, in terms of the share of Government Insurance in the financing of China's urban health care system, see table 6.3). Employees of government, public agency, and state-owned enterprise were worse off, however, in terms of conditions of medical treatment. Nevertheless, the new medical insurance had a good budget, which indicates its sustainability in the longer term; there might be some advances in horizontal equity, and even vertical equity, as co-payment ratios are relatively light and reimbursement conditions are being liberalized. Placing these advancements in the larger context of national health costs, in both absolute and relative terms, it is clear that enormous resources were put into a system that turned out to be very inequitable by comparison with other nations. In other words, the advancements of the health care reform did not mitigate this scenario—an inequitable health care financing structure is firmly in place, institutionalized by the new health care reform initiatives, despite the many advances of the new system in terms of cost reduction and quality improvement.

It should be noted that this chapter confines itself to examining the central question of whether health care reform, and the full implementation of Basic Health Insurance, in particular, has advanced in terms of equity. There are many other equally important health care issues in China. For instance, on the cost-efficiency side, health care reform has been much more successful. But there are areas outside medical insurance, such as preventive health care—an area in which the SARS outbreaks in 2003 and 2004 revealed problems—that demand urgent government intervention. We also have not directly addressed the issue of quality of health care per se but the question of equitable access to quality health care at a basic level. Moreover, regional disparities in health care are a growing concern, in view of the widening income gap between the coastal provinces and the western and northeastern regions on one hand, and between the cities and the rural areas on the other. These are important issues in their own right, though they are not the focus of the present discussion.

Notes

1. Jun Gao. et al., "Changing Access to Health Services in Urban China: Implications for Equity," *Health Policy and Planning* 16, no. 3 (2001): 302–312; Colleen M. Grogan, "Urban Economic Reform and Access to Health Care Coverage in the People's Republic of China," *Social Science and Medicine* 41, no. 8 (1995): 1073–84; Gordon G. Liu, et al., "Equity in Health Care Access: Assessing the Urban Health Insurance Reform in China," *Social Science and Medicine* 55, no. 10 (November, 2002): 1779–1794; Xing-zhu Liu and William C.L.Hsiao, "The Cost Escalation of Social Health Insurance Plans in China: Its Implication for Public Policy," *Social Science and Medicine* 41, no. 8 (1995): 1095–1101; Yuan-li Liu, William C. Hsiao and Karen Eggleston, "Equity in Health and Health Care: the Chinese Experience," *Social Science and Medicine* 49, no. 10 (November, 1999): 1349– 1356.

2. Grogan, (1995), 1073, for example, on a person's place of employment as the basis for distribution health care benefits.

3. There is clearly the case for explaining the lack of health care protection for migrant workers who do not have urban household registration status. Recently, the government under the Premier Wan appeared to take note of this rural-urban divide and pledged to work on it.

4. Gao. et al., (2001), 302–312; Grogan, (1995), 1073–84; Hong Wang and Chun-guang Wang, "Some Thoughts about Building the Basic Medical Protection System for the Poor People in City and Towns," *Labor Protection World* no. 2 (2003): 18–20 (in Chinese); Hui-lin Zhuan, "Urban Deprived Groups in the New Era: Studying the Construction of a Health Care Protection Mechanism," *Market and Population Analysis* (May 23, 2003): 23–28 (in Chinese).

5. Xin-ping Guan, "Poverty and Antipoverty Policies in Urban China." in *Poverty Monitoring and Alleviation in East Asia*, ed. Kwong-leung Tang and Chack-kie Wong (New York: Nova Science Press, 2003), 15–37.

6. Zhuan, (2003), 18–19.

7. Zhuan, (2003), 20. In 2002, China had a population of 19.98 million urban poor whowere classified as having an average household income less than the official poverty relief standard, which varies according to cities but is higher than the national poverty line for the rural poor, which sets at the subsistence level. The monetary value is now at an average income of 637 yuan, recently released by the Poverty Eradication Office of the State Council, reported by the *Hong Kong Economic Journal* 30 July 2004.

8. They are referred to the urban poor who do not have either medical insurance or medical assistance. Source: Zhong-xiang Liu, " A Study of the Problem Related to Medical Assistance for Urban Poor," (Unpublished manuscript. Sociology Department, the People's University of China, 2003), Table 2 (in Chinese).

9. Gini Cofficient is measured in terms of 0=absolute equality, 1=absolute inequality. Usually 0.4 is regarded as the threshold of serious inequality in income inequality measure. Source: Pei-lin Li, "Problems and Trends of China's Social and Economic Developments." http://china.com.cn/chinese/zhuanti/2004shxs/483054.htm (accessed 17 January 2004).

10. *Ibid.* Liu, et al., (2002).

11. Article 6 of the "Notice Concerning the Temporary Control in the Use of Drugs of City and Township Employees under Basic Medical Insurance," *Ministry of Labor and Social Security* no. 15 (12 May 1999) (in Chinese).

12. *See* Appendix to the "Notice Concerning the Management of Consultation Items of City and Township Employee under Basic Medical Insurance." *Ministry of Labor and Social Security* no. 44 (30 June 1999) (in Chinese).

13. For example, according to the Medical Insurance Bureau of Zhengjiang City, the annual increase rate of total health care expense for employees had decreased from 33.4 percent in pre-reform era to 16.3 percent afterward. Source: Zhenjiang Insurance Bureau, "Zhenjiang Health Care Reform," www.zjyb.gov.cn/ybjj/htm (accessed 6 September 2002) (in Chinese). Also see Gordon G. Liu, et al., "Urban Health Care Reform Initiative in China: Findings from its Pilot Experiment in Zhenjiang City," *International Journal of Economic Development* 4 (1999): 504–526.

14. Ministry of Health, *Brief Report of the Development of Health Affairs in China, 1997–2001*. (2001), www.moh.gov.cn/tjxxzx/tjsj/tjgbl/200304030003.htm (accessed 23 January 2003) (in Chinese).

15. Calculation based on figures available from China National Statistical Bureau: 523,760 thousand for urban population and 256,390 thousand for urban labor force.

16. Cross-tabulation on the basis of statement of income and expenditure of the Hospital Authority, "Hong Kong, Annual Report of Hospital Authority, 2002–2003," www.ha-org.hk (accessed 17 January 2004).

17. Wei Yu, "The Important Issue of Enterprise Reform: Health Care Insurance System." in *The Reformability of China's State Sector*, ed. G. J. Wen and D. Xu (Singapore: World Scientific,1997).

18. Po-guang Hsia, "Enthusiastic Discussion of Medical Care Protection by Representatives," *China Social Security System* 4 (2003): 20–23; Jian-feng Bai, "What Does Medical Reform Bring?" *Renmin Ribao*, 12 January 2001 (in Chinese).

19. Ministry of Health, *An Analysis Report of the Secondary National Health Survey, 1998*. (July 1999), www.moh.gov.cn/statistics/ronhs98/ronhs41.doc (accessed 23 January 2003) (in Chinese).

20. Wuhan Municipal Government, "The City Conditions of Wuhan," www.whtj.gov.cn/whsq/shsq2004/index.htm (accessed 5 September 2004) (in Chinese).

21. World Health Organization, *World Health Report 2000—Health System: Improving Performance*, (Geneva:WHO, 2000), 4. www.who.int/whr2001.2001/archives/2000/en/index.htm (accessed 5 August 2004).

22. *Ibid*., Annex Table 1.

23. William C. L. Hsiao, "The Chinese Health Care System: Lessons for Other Nations," *Social Science and Medicine* 41, no. 8 (1995): 1047–1055, 1047; World Bank, *China: Long-Term Issues and Options in the Health Transition* (Washington, D.C.: World Bank, 1992), xi.

Chapter 7

Going Down the Road of Developmentalism: The Future of the Health Care System in China

Following its establishment in 1949, Communist China developed a unique health services system, characterized by decentralization, continuity with traditional medicine, integration with the local political structure, and mass participation.[1] In the urban areas, health care was financed by the work unit or employer. Before economic reform in 1980, government funding covered the full costs of public health institutions, and patients were charged fee-for-service in accordance with a centrally planned national fee schedule.[2]

Academics have pointed to some important achievements made by China in social welfare provision, including the ideology of equity for all citizens and the near universal availability of adequate food, education, housing, jobs, transport, and accessible and affordable treatment and preventive health services.[3] A cursory overview of the current state of the health care system in China prompts the following observation: With limited resources, China has probably developed the world's largest network of health care services, and the health status of its people has risen dramatically during the past forty years. Even the poorest sections of the population have had their health needs met.

It is now common knowledge that China's economic transformation from a communist centrally planned economy to a market-oriented economy was carried out under the leadership of Deng Xiao-ping. Economic reform in China started in 1978, and its impact quickly spilled over to other policy arenas, including health care. As Hu[4] points out, the restructuring of China's health insurance in urban areas was in line with the requirements of the general reform of the economic system. As part of the social security reforms, China's health care system has been undergoing major changes since the early 1980s.[5]

As discussed in chapters 2 and 3, the transformation of China's health care system has taken place in the wake of the changes in economic policy, marked by fiscal and service decentralization. The area of health provision has seen such important changes as the disintegration of the rural cooperative medical service, the decentralization of township hospitals from county to township governments, the requirement of official permission for private practice, the implementation of a personal responsibility system in health institutions, the reform of health security, and the introduction of health insurance in rural areas.[6] In short, health delivery in post-1978 China has been marked by reduced government funding as well as an ideology of a reduced government role in the financing and provision of health services. In 1995, health care spending accounted for only some 17 percent of total government spending (see table 6.6). In the same period, the government's budget for health contributed only some 10 to 15 percent of total hospital expenditures, barely covering the salaries of health workers.

As a result, fiscal stringency has forced most hospitals to seek revenue from other sources, for example, charging above-cost prices for high-technology diagnostic procedures and using the excess to cross-subsidize services that were priced below cost.[7] Numerous studies have shown the adverse impact of government budgetary controls. Zheng and Hillier[8] studied the effects of Chinese health care reform on hospitals in the middle-income counties of Jiangxi Province. They found that hospitals without state subsidies were making up for their revenue shortfall by increased medicine sales and economic targeting by individual hospital departments. Even the traditional Chinese medical institutions have had to rely increasingly on medicine sales for revenue, and they have still been operating at a deficit.

All of this has led to escalating health costs. As noted in previous chapters, the pilot health insurance reform began in Zhenjiang and Jiujiang cities in 1994, to counter the problems of cost escalation and financial sustainability. The experiment was extended in 1996 to fifty-seven other cities, and finally, at the end of 1998, it went nationwide.

The Reformed Urban Health Care System: Pros and Cons

As noted, several key features can be found in the reformed urban health system: personal medical accounts, out-of-pocket spending by beneficiaries in the form of deductibles and co-insurance, and social risk pooling at the city level. Undoubtedly, this reform had great policy significance, with important implications for China and other East Asian countries. A decade after the pilot health insurance reform, academics and policy makers in China and overseas are eager to know whether it has worked thus far.

Using four criteria (i.e., coverage, consumer choice, portability, cost control), this study finds that the new health care system has certain merits. Undoubtedly, more people in the urban areas now gain access to health care services following the health care reform. The current Basic Health Insurance scheme is intended to cover all urban employers and employees, and all enterprises, state administrative departments, institutions and other organizations, and their staff members and workers are obliged to pay the basic medical insurance premiums. Further, the medical insurance program gives patients a choice of doctor and provides for portability of benefits. This provision is particularly important to the economic development of China as labor mobility is enhanced by the ability of workers to carry their benefits from one place to another. As the central government has taken over from enterprises the responsibility for health insurance, collectivism has been partially preserved through redistributory "risk-pooling."[9] Last but not least, the Basic Health Insurance scheme has partially controlled escalating health costs, stabilizing the rising trend of health spending.

In sum, the new health care system has achieved some of its goals. Relying on a mix of social risk pooling and personal accounts, the new system is better than the former health system, which benefited only selected groups of enterprise workers and government officials and their family members. Judged against the goals laid out in the health care reform, which include wider coverage and containment of costs, it is clear that the medical insurance program has made significant headway. The financial sustainability of the system has been enhanced, and the administrative costs of running the new health system are not exorbitant.

Empirical studies of the reformed health system have identified both its strengths and weaknesses. Some of the positive achievements noted in the literature echo those discussed earlier. For instance, evidence collected by overseas scholars after the early stage of reform showed that these measures were successful in reducing real per capita health care expenditure, and there were reductions in length of stay and in the prescription of expensive diagnostic tests.[10]

A later but more extensive study conducted by Liu and his associates[11] found some positive changes in access to health care in the wake of the pilot experiment with the urban health insurance reform. Specifically, their study examined the pre- and post-reform changes in the likelihood of obtaining various health care services across subpopulation groups with different socioeconomic statuses and health conditions.

Relying upon data from the annual surveys conducted in Zhenjiang City (1994– 96), their study showed that there was significant horizontal inequity before the health insurance reform: The likelihood of obtaining basic care in the outpatient setting was much higher for those with higher income, education, and job status. Importantly, however, there was no evidence suggesting vertical inequity against people with chronic disease conditions in access to care in various settings. After the health care reform, Liu and his associates[12] found that the new insurance led to a significant increase in the uptake on outpatient care by the lower socioeconomic groups, resulting in horizontal equity in access to basic care. The new insurance plan also maintained a measure of vertical equity in the use of all types of care. Overall, Liu et al.[13] demonstrated that the health reform resulted in improved equity in access to basic care provided in outpatient settings. There was some evidence pointing to greater efficiency in the allocation of health care resources since outpatient care now took the place of more expensive care in emergency or inpatient settings.

Where the weakness of the health care system becomes apparent is in the plight of the uninsured. More important, the new program compares badly with those in other countries. Government spending on health as a share of total spending in China has dwindled from 36.2 percent in the early 1980s to 15 percent in 2002. In terms of the fairness of the system of financial contributions to the costs of health, China was ranked near the bottom of the league by the WHO in 2000.

Some empirical studies also highlight deficiencies in the reformed program. According to Liu and Mills, for instance, while market-oriented reforms in health care have improved the productivity of public health institutions, they have brought about some significant unintended consequences: the overprovision of unnecessary services and the underprovision of socially desirable services; the reduction in the take-up of preventive services after the introduction of user fees; and the underprovision of services with public goods characteristics.[14]

Other studies of the reformed health care system in China are decidedly more pessimistic. For instance, an empirical study conducted by Duckett[15] in Tianjin, Suzhou, Beijing, and Shanghai gave a sanguine view of the development of health care reform in China. She found that urban health reform policy has been implemented slowly. Local health insurance schemes have suffered from poor participation rates. There have also been difficulties balancing contributions to local government-run pooled funds with the expenditures needed for medical treatment. She contended that the main problems with the reformed health schemes are due to the vested interests of the various parties—enterprises, hospitals, and officials—who had been the beneficiaries of the pre-reform system.

Duckett[16] found that decentralization of social services led local governments in China to set up new ways to fund their work. This produced variable quality in welfare health within localities and further fragmented the state. Local governments often found it difficult to force state enterprises to participate in health insurance schemes if they were ranked at the same or a higher level. Worse, there was no legislation requiring enterprise participation. Duckett thus cautioned that unless something is done, these problems will threaten the viability of the national program.

Duckett's[17] observations regarding decentralization, fragmentation, and the locus of authority merit some scrutiny. As noted in chapter 3, it is true that the progress of China's health insurance reform is unbalanced: Some cities are over-insured while others are still struggling to establish a socially pooled fund and personal medical accounts. However, there is some evidence that the local schemes are converging, in terms of both theory and practice, toward the system envisioned by the State Council. In this regard, the Decision concerning the Establishment of the Basic Health Insurance System for Urban Staff and Workers, promulgated by the State Council in 1998, has helped to build some uniformity across programs. Following this decree, the labor insurance health system and publicly funded health system were unified into the Basic Health Insurance System for Urban Staff and Workers. In essence, the 1998 Decree sets out some general principles and an implementation framework for the provincial, municipal, and autonomous regional governments to follow. Thus, there is reason to believe that many of the problems identified by Duckett have been addressed following the proclamation of the Decree.

As of today, the reforms in the financing of China's public health services are characterized by a reduction in government budgetary support and the introduction of charges. Admittedly, health resources and service utilization in urban areas are still much greater than in the rural regions. Despite this, there is a downside: People with poor socioeconomic status continue to be disadvantaged in accessing expensive and advanced diagnostic technologies. One would guess that in the context of a rapidly growing aged population, market-driven health services would disadvantage certain categories of people in the urban areas: *xiagang* workers, older people, and the poor as well as the chronically ill. Added to this list are the disabled, the floating population (migrants), and the uninsured.

Several selected groups seem to be the losers under the new health care scheme. An empirical study conducted by Gao and his associates[18]reviewed health care utilization among different income groups in China. This study made use of data from the national health surveys conducted in 1993 and 1998, covering some 16,000 households and 54,000 individuals in the urban areas. The findings showed a significant decline in the population covered by Government Insurance and Labor Insurance, while the proportion of the population who had to pay for services out of pocket increased from 28 percent in 1993 to 44.1 percent in 1998 (rising further to 44.8 in 2003, see table 6.3). They found that more people who reported illness from each income group received medical treatment of some kind, but there was a decline in seeking care from a health provider.

Overall, Gao and his associates[19] found that access to health care by the urban population has become more inequitable. The unemployed face increasing difficulties in accessing health care. The poor, likewise, face many difficulties. Among those in the lowest income group who, in 1998, reported illness but did not obtain treatment of any kind, nearly 70 percent (as compared with 38 percent in 1993) claimed financial difficulty as the major reason. The use of inpatient services dropped significantly from 4.5 percent in 1993 to 3.0 percent in 1998.

The decreased use of inpatient services was more serious in the lowest and lower income groups than in the higher and highest income groups. The percentage of patients who were referred for hospital admission but were not hospitalized had a negative relationship with income level.

Current Urban Health Care Program

This cursory review of the literature shows that it is important to find ways to deal with the challenges raised. The emerging health care system in China needs some serious restructuring. Before we set out our views on the future of health care delivery in China, it is important to capture all the essential features of the current health care system.

Overall, how would one characterize the reformed urban health care delivery in China? At the macro level, China's transition to a socialist market economy has brought decreased reliance on state funding, decentralization of public health services, increased autonomy of health facilities, increased freedom of movement of health workers, decreased political control, and changes in rural health services.[20]

The current urban health care model is characterized by multiple players (i.e., governments [central and local], employers, employees, etc.), multiple financing sources, and the support of all kinds of complementary health insurance programs.[21] This model is clearly not socialist, either in orientation or in practice. Health care in present-day China is no longer a state-provided public service. There is no nationalized health care system for all. With the emphasis on individual responsibility (through the setting up of personal medical accounts), the government is attempting to take a back seat in health care delivery.

Neither is the current path of health reform neo-liberal, since health care in China is certainly not seen as an item of personal consumption and a large portion of the population remains poor. Furthermore, despite the introduction of a user-fee system and the dwindling financial role of the central government, the market is not dominant in the health care system in China. Thus, even while it sheds all responsibility for health care provision, the central government maintains its strong regulatory role in health care.

Overall, we believe that the current practice reflects a pluralistic health care model.[22] The reformed system clearly places increased financial responsibility on the insured persons (contributions and benefit structure) coupled with reduced levels of benefit. In other words, individuals and their families are urged to shoulder more of the financial burden of health care. Further, the introduction of personal medical accounts demonstrates the importance given to self-reliance, while the collective socially pooled fund illustrates the importance attached to social insurance principles.[23] Should these two accounts fail to provide for health expenses, then supplemental insurance programs would kick in, including the state-financed complementary scheme (for civil servants), non-profit schemes, and commercial schemes. In other words, the present reformed system is built on a plurality of financing sources. Multiple players are involved: individuals, families, enterprises, local government, central government, and the non-profit as well as the for-profit sector. Their complementary contributions are intended to make the whole system work.

Alternative Policy Options

What are the prospects for continued reform and progress in the future? There are an array of options for China, ranging from the neo-liberal to the pluralistic, from the socialist to the developmentalist.

First of all, there have been calls for a privatized health care system in China, mainly from the neo-liberal camp. They argue that continued market growth in China would create this acceptable alternative to the current reform. Can China afford to go down this route? Given the current level of economic development, many urban people in China are unable to finance their own health care, and a privatized system would in the end worsen existing income inequities between the well off and the poor and between urban and rural people. The for-profit sector tends to target the rich and the insured and specializes in services that can be sold to the well off for high prices.[24]

Believing that reliance on government should not be the sole source of funding for health care, the World Bank[25] argues in favor of introducing user fees and some form of health insurance. Thus, it supports market-oriented health care reform in China. However, realizing that there are some inadequacies in this approach, based on the experience in the Third World, the World Bank Report[26] on health financing in China offered the following series of recommendations, suggesting appropriate measures to deal with privatization and shortage of public resources:

- Greater emphasis on primary care
- Reductions in hospitalization
- Improvement in quality of personnel
- Greater focus on cost effectiveness
- Higher quality of health care management

One could draw some useful lessons from the "privatization" of China's rural health care since the early 1980s. Following fiscal devolution, the rural primary health service was transformed into a fee-for-service system, dependent on the availability of local resources. A recent study by Kaufman and Fang[27] reported the impact of privatization on financing, provision, and the use of reproductive health services by women in two rural counties in Yunnan Province. They found that the most common self-reported symptoms of reproductive morbidity were abnormal vaginal discharge and vaginal tears during home delivery, which went mostly untreated. Very little use was made of hospital-based delivery and prenatal care because of the high costs and the perceived low quality of these services. Service quality was affected by low investment in training, maintenance, and supervision of workers. Most of the burden for maternal and child health care fell on local health workers, yet the latter's resources had been declining from 1985 to 1995. In short, researchers found that rural women's reproductive health needs were inadequately attended to by rural health services following the health care reforms in the rural areas.

More recently, Peter Lindert, in his book, *Growing Public*, argues, "The gains from offering universal benefits, instead of tight means testing, are most obvious in the realm of public health and health insurance. The more privatized U.S. health system is more bureaucratic, plagued by incentive problems, moreunequally distributed and less successful in saving lives."[28] Even the World Bank in their publication *Financing Health Care: Issues and Options for China* categorically rejects this approach. It states in the very beginning that "Health is a sector that cannot simply be left to the market forces."[29]

A privatized health care system is often proposed as the alternative to a system provided wholly by the state, as demonstrated in the quote from Lindert. As a matter of fact, many people were worried over China's situation in the wake of its World Trade Organization (WTO) entry. There are some concerns that the WTO might demand that the Chinese privatize and deregulate the health sector.[30] Even as China moves away from a centrally planned economy and toward a market-based approach, there have been some voices in favor of a stronger (and exclusive) role of the state. Researchers have affirmed the positive impacts of universal health care delivery. This approach is couched in terms of rights. A right-based approach emphasizes universal and adequate health protection for all people. It emphasizes the need for government intervention and the importance of comprehensive social programs that will not only provide a comprehensive safety net but also actively promote the welfare of all.

This state-led approach appeals to some people in China. For instance, academics like Ho and Tsai praised the publicly funded health care system that existed under Mao:

> Under Chairman Mao Zedong, more than 90 percent of the population of China enjoyed government-subsidized cradle-to-grave health care. Those living in cities received more comprehensive coverage from hospitals, while the rural dwellers primarily sought medical attention from "barefoot doctors" and local clinics. . . . The government used funds from farming collectives to pay for rural doctors and clinics. Although this system provided only basic care, such initiatives helped double life expectancy in China to sixty-five years by the mid-1970s. In comparison to other developing countries such as India, Burma, Vietnam, and North Korea, China's health care system was far more effective and was often held up as a shining example to the rest of the

developing world.[31]

It is hard to envisage China going back to the socialist model in health care provision. First, it would impose a great financial burden on China. China simply could not financially support a system built on free and universal health care for all citizens. Second, such an approach is not congruent with the dominant trend of the socialist market system, which emphasizes individual responsibility.

In the same vein, the present pluralist model is marked by a number of significant flaws, as revealed in our empirical study. Our survey and other studies demonstrate that the existing health system has many limitations. The dwindling role of the government is a cause for concern in the eyes of the respondents in Wuhan. The Chinese government would be ill advised to do no more than maintain the status quo.

We are not alone in criticizing the present health system. Duckett, for instance, argues that the medical insurance scheme has many problems arising from the vested interests of those enterprises, hospitals, officials, health service providers, producers of medicines, enterprise employees, and enterprise managers who benefited from the pre-reform system.[32] These people "have sought to resist changes that erode their benefits or damage their interests."[33] The policy reforms have thus been implemented slowly, and local health insurance schemes have had difficulties balancing the contributions to local government-run socially pooled funds with the amounts they have had to pay out for medical treatment. She notes that most health insurance schemes have had problems with financing their socially pooled funds that were used to pay for treatment. Inevitably, rising medical costs will pose problems for these schemes. It has to be pointed out that as the health care reform continues, a rising surplus in the reserves pool would help alleviate the financial constraints faced by the local government.

Relevance of Developmentalism

Despite the visible achievements, China faces a number of challenges in its health care reform. To recapitulate, some of the key findings of our study are summarized as follows:

(1) The respondents were generally in favor of health care reform emphasizing a policy shift from collective to individual responsibility in health care protection.

(2) Nearly two-thirds of respondents agreed that it was reasonable for an individual to bear part of the medical expenses. It seems that the mix of a socially pooled fund for redistribution and personal medical accounts is acceptable to most employee respondents.

(3) The respondents endorsed the three main components of health care

reform —in particular, the Basic Health Insurance. The old ethos in which the state is seen as primarily responsible for basic health care protection appealed to them.

(4) An overwhelming majority of respondents regarded the government or the employment units as having the major responsibility for assisting those who were unable to pay for medical fees.

(5) High medical expenses are a burden to our respondents. Not consulting doctors was found to be a common practice. An overwhelming majority of respondents were particularly worried about medical expenses in case of serious illness.

(6) Only some 21 percent of the total urban population, or 31 percent of the total urban working population, are covered by health insurance in Wuhan. Thus, the health needs of the overwhelming majority in the urban area were not protected by the health insurance schemes.

(7) As far as health care financing is concerned, the role played by the state has been reduced significantly.

Three groups of stakeholders were interviewed through focus groups in January 2004, subsequent to the surveys in Wuhan (the groups comprised seven insured people from enterprise, a group of five officials from the social insurance center, and a group of six personnel from two medical establishments). Overall, their views were not unanimous.

The first focus group expressed some concerns about the current reform: delays in treatment and limited choice of hospitals. Some interviewees felt that they were now being treated unequally, unlike in the past. Another questioned the dwindling role of t he government. Their general sentiment was that the state was uncaring when it came to health care provision. In contrast with these views, the respondents from among the officials expressed positive feelings toward the reform. Some of them argued that medical insurance was important to economic development and social stability. Also, it gave more protection to the people.

Finally, the attitudes of those medical personnel that we spoke to were more ambivalent. In particular, they pointed out that serious and chronic illnesses were still a problem for vulnerable groups in society. They pointed to those people who were not covered by the new medical insurance. Some problems were noted, including the view that co-payments were fairly low. However, they were optimistic about the future development of medical insurance. One hospital administrator opined that when more enterprises joined the new medical insurance, more patients would benefit.

Taking all these findings into account, it is clear that there is scant support for the privatization of health care in China. The need for change is obvious, and the government cannot afford to change the health care system incrementally. More important, the central government would have to formulate a solution to close the gap between those with and without health care in urban areas. In our survey findings, there is some support for developmentalism, which favors increased government intervention in the health services and the provision of universal services for the citizens (i.e., health for all), while ensuring such services are compatible with economic development.

In our study, the respondents generally endorse the principle tenet of developmentalism: The state has a key role in harmonizing social and economic development. The respondents generally think that the present model of medical expenses is problematic because the state does not contribute its share in the financing of health insurance, while the general public cannot afford expensive health care services and medication. A majority of our respondents are worried about their future health care protection. Clearly, in the eyes of our survey respondents, the central government should not abrogate its financial responsibilities in health care. The continued involvement of the Chinese government in the system represents a pragmatic approach to dealing with the health care issue.

There is now a compelling case for increased state spending in health insurance programs.[34] We note in chapter 6 that the central government in China has played a dwindling role in overall social security provision. Until now, the Chinese government has continued to reduce its expenditure on health care (relative to total government spending). Clearly, based on our findings, the central government should not be doing this but should reverse this worrying trend. With the rapid economic growth of the past two decades, China is in the financial position to invest more in health care provision. With the gradual reform of the taxation system, the fiscal power of the central government will be enhanced, and it will be in a better position to fund health care.

Such an increase in health care financing is congruent with the WHO's recommendation. According to the WHO,[35] high-income countries (those with a per capita income [at current prices] above US$8,000 per annum), on average, spend 8 percent of national income on health (annual health spending ranges from US$1000 to more than US$4,000 per capita). In middle-income countries (those with per capita income between US$1,000 and US$8,000), between 3 percent and 7 percent of national income is spent on health, representing an annual expenditure of between US$75 and US$550 per capita. Finally, low-income countries (those with annual per capita income of less than US$ 1,000) are deficient in resources and can spend only 1 to 3 percent of GDP on health.

Since China's GDP (at current prices) in 2003 has passed the level of US$1,000 (the alternative measure being US$4,020, based on PPP),[36] it can aim to spend 3 to 7 percent of national income on health care. Such an increase is congruent with the principle tenets of developmentalism. There should be a corresponding increase in the share of health spending from the government budget. The 1990 level could be used as a point of reference, that is, some 25 percent of total government spending could be spent on health care (see table 6.6). This would help relieve the pressure on cities, prefectures, and counties to find the money to make up the gap between subsidies and actual spending.

Unlike the pluralistic approach, developmentalism rejects the call for the abolition of state welfare and calls for a stronger role of the state, which is relevant to the context of reform China. The historical concern of developmentalism with social welfare is compatible with the rights-based, social protection approach. While developmentalism transcends the limitations of this rights-based approach, it promotes the goals of social protection and the notion of social rights in ways that may be meaningful to the East Asian nations. As discussed in chapter 4, the theory of developmentalism embraces the following policy options: investment in human capital, investment in asset development, investment in social capital, removal of barriers to economic participation, and investment in employment programs.

Drawing on these principles, the proponents of developmentalism call for policy changes that would extend the coverage of health insurance to workers in private enterprises and foreign-owned enterprises.[37] More important, they see the change toward health insurance with personal medical accounts in China as a step in the right direction. It serves to promote individual responsibility. Through their contributions, workers are taking care of their future. The use of personal medical accounts overcomes the disadvantage of the old system that benefits only a few selected groups. In our findings, respondents generally endorse out-of-pocket payments for health care beyond basic levels. Hence, the setting up of personal medical savings accounts should not be seen as equivalent to full privatization of health care, as the full swing of the market is yet to come in the case of China. Rather, such personal accounts should be seen as individual contributions to their health needs, as a form of asset building for future use.[38]

In the view of developmentalism, the implementation of basic medical insurance is desirable as, in essence, it provides a basic floor of health protection to the people. The government has the responsibility to provide free basic health care. Furthermore, the reformed health system provides for social risk pooling, which is the correct thing to do.[39] By pooling together all individual workers' and enterprises' contributions, the contributions collected from workers can be used to finance the claims of unhealthy workers. Obviously, more work can be done in this area in the future: city-level pooling funds, unification of the contribution rate as a proportion of payrolls, and the payment of benefits and the collection of contributions in full.

According to developmentalist thinking, the Chinese government should change its mind-set, seeing health care provision as a productivist social policy and program. It should transcend the remedial and maintenance preoccupations of conventional welfarist approaches and, instead, seek to invest in the capabilities of needy people to participate effectively in the productive economy. In this approach, social expenditure on health care ceases to become costly benefit transfers but investments that generate a return to the economy and to society as a whole.

Obviously, increasing government spending on health care is not enough. The present health care system leaves room for improvement in the areas of drug dispensing, price, and payment reforms as well as provisions for the uninsured. First and foremost, to discourage health care providers from the excessive prescribing and selling of drugs, the government needs to unlink health providers' revenue from drug sales by separating the drug prescription from the dispensing function.

Moreover, necessary price and payment reforms must be instituted, with the objectives of controling costs while ensuring access to patients and allowing hospitals to sustain themselves financially.[40] As discussed in Bitran and Yip[41], Shanghai conducted a successful experiment to contain hospital costs. Facing a substantial increase in hospital costs from 1993 to 1994, Shanghai instituted a global hospital budget system: Hospital costs were permitted to increase no more than 24 percent, and drugs were held to a 15-percent maximum increase. Fees for visits and surgeries were reduced to align them with the labor costs involved, and fees for MRI and CT services were reduced by 12 to 15 percent.

The current health care system leaves millions of people uninsured. Yip and Hsiao observe:

> The current reform policies segment the urban health sector into a number of subsectors, but there are no coherent pricing and payment policies across these segmented but interrelated sectors. The financing reform distinctly creates two separate groups among the urban population: the insured and the uninsured. Among the insured, there are two separate service markets: services covered under the social insurance scheme, and services not covered. Among the uninsured, economic transition further creates two subpopulations: the high- and the low-income.[42]

Those uninsured people with low income have not received much attention from officials. There must be measures to help those who are not insured (i.e., those people at the periphery of the health reform). For instance, the setting up of special designated funds will help. Some pioneering projects like the one in the Shenzhen plan to set up a designated fund for the uninsured (*Interview with Shenzhen's Social Security Bureau Head, 19 November 2003*). The role of the central government is important, as it must take the lead in formulating comprehensive policies to deal with the issue in the long run.

Conclusion

It should be noted that international organizations and academics have suggested other remedies targeting specific problems encountered in the health reform. Thus the WHO[43] calls for the reinforcement of health systems to be based on the core principles of primary health care as outlined at Alma-Ata in 1978: universal access and coverage on the basis of need; health equity as part of development oriented to social justice; community participation in defining and implementing health agendas; and intersectoral approaches to health. These principles hold true for China. At the same time, while they provide a broad vision that is valid for all countries, their detailed implementation has yet to be worked out in China.

Academics and policy analysts also offer their recommendations. Duckett[44] contends that the introduction of national health insurance legislation and better monitoring and regulation of enterprises and hospitals is indispensable. Despite these measures, Duckett was not optimistic, as she observed that citizens' voices in China are not strong. She concluded by saying: "The difficulties attached to remedying these fundamental problems (i.e., weak local government capacity) mean that interests (i.e., enterprise, hospital, individual interests) created in the pre-re-form Mao era will continue to dominate health insurance reform."[45] As noted earlier, the 1998 Decree issued by the central government represents a significant directive that aims at addressing the issues of monitoring and implementation, and it has thus gone some way to addressing the criticisms of Duckett.

On the future of health care reform, a rather cautious assessment comes from Cheung and Gu, who pay much attention to the potential impact of economic growth:

> The prospect of such [health] reform depends very much on an effective containment of medical expenditure, as well as economic growth that can improve the ability to pay of the working population. In the meantime, the reduction in insurance coverage has left many urban poor and less-protected rural families more vulnerable.[46]

Inevitably, economic growth and cost containment can only partially answer the question. We believe that a macro normative framework that ties economic development with social development is needed urgently. In this regard, the normative theory of developmentalism would be most relevant to China's health reform.

The World Summit on Social Development, which was held in Copenhagen in 1995, has popularized the idea of social development that serves as a counter to neo-liberal principles.[47] This approach gives expression to two axioms: First, it requires that economic development should be inclusive, integrated, and sustainable and that it should bring benefits to all; and second, it proposes that social welfare should be investment oriented, seeking to enhance human capacities to participate in the productive economy. This approach offers a perspective that may facilitate a renewed basis for state intervention in health care in the case of China.

The central notion of the social development approach is the concern with the total population. It is therefore inclusive in scope, a major focus being the needy and poor. It calls for a minimum floor of social protection for all citizens while acknowledging the importance of individual responsibility. More important, it supports increased people's participation in the determination of both the means and outcome of development.

In this regard, we contend that developmentalism should form a central and normative framework for the central government. The central government should go down the route of developmentalism to ensure that social policies and programs contribute positively to development, without creating conditions of welfare dependency and without harming economic growth. In this regard, China should build on the country's tradition of intervention to urge policy makers to actively address social concerns like health care needs.

More important, this recommendation is congruent with the findings of health studies[48] that the Chinese experience in health care reform would generate important lessons: A decline in the role of government in financing public health services is likely to result in decreased overall efficiency of the health sector. Importantly, as Liu and Mills rightly argue, levying charges for public health services can reduce demand for these services and increase the risk of disease transmission.

Overall, if China adopts the approach of developmentalism, it will have the following strengths. First, this approach calls for a closer integration of social and economic policies to promote *welfare for all*. It is consistent with the "Five Coordinations" as advanced by Hu Jin-tao, the Communist Party chairman. Advocates of the developmental approach urge the adoption of macroeconomic policies that promote employment and attain people-centred economic development outcomes. To achieve this goal, investment in human capital is critical. A sound health system would ensure that the workers enter, and participate effectively in, the productive economy.[49] A health care system that is inclusive of all is critically important in the case of China. As noted in earlier chapters, the plight of the marginalized people excluded from the health care system deserves utmost attention from the Chinese leaders. Their exclusion calls for more state intervention, particularly in the financing of health care provision. Increased state intervention is paralleled by an acknowledgment of individual responsibility in the provision of social services, as most nations in contemporary contexts have found it impossible to supply free and universal services for all citizens without levying heavy taxation.

Further, developmentalism promotes a pluralistic approach to social welfare that transcends the historic welfare statism of the European nations. Recognizing that the state cannot, and indeed should not, assume sole responsibility for economic development and social welfare, social developmentalism urges the integrated involvement of the state, the market, and the community. Known as the institutional approach to social development, it proposes that governments direct the process of social development in ways that maximize the participation of communities, markets, and individuals in both economic and social development. This approach should appeal to the Chinese government, which has effectively exercised state direction over economic development but has not dismissed the contribution of the market, the community, and popular participation.

Finally, the theory of developmental welfare promotes a consensual development model. The major stakeholders involved in promoting social development include the state, the community, non-governmental organizations, employers, and workers. By involving many constituencies in both economic and social policy, the prospects for reviving solidarity and promoting social integration increase. In an increasingly unequal society like China, the goal of promoting social integration should be given high priority.

Notes

1. J. G. Andersen, "Health Care in the People's Republic of China: A Blend of Traditional and Modern," *Central Issues in Anthropology* 10 (1992): 67–75.

2. Ricardo Bitran and Winnie C. Yip, "A Review of Health Care Provider Payment Reform in Selected Countries in Asia and Latin America," (Major Applied Research 2, Working Paper 1, Bethesda, Maryland: Partnerships for Health Reform Project, Abt Associates, August 1998).

3. Pel-lin Yang, Vivian Lin and James Lawson, "Health Policy Reform in the People's Republic of China," *International Journal of Health Services* 21, no. 3 (1991): 481–491.

4. Zu-liu Hu, "Social Protection and Enterprise Reform," in *Enterprise and Social Benefits from Communism*, ed. M. Rein, B. Friedman and A. Worgotter (Cambridge: Cambridge University Press, 1998), 284–304.

5. Russell Smyth, "Labor-Market and Social-Welfare Reform in the State-Owned Sector in China," *Journal of Developing Areas* 33, no. 2 (1999): 223–244.

6. Xing-zhu Liu and J. L. Wang, "An Introduction to China's Health Care System," *Journal of Public Health Policy* 2, no. 1 (1991): 104–116.

7. Bitran and Yip, (1998).

8. Xiang Zheng and Sheila Hillier, "The Reforms of the Chinese Health Care System:County Level Changes: The Jiangxi Study," *Social Science and Medicine* 41, no. 8 (1995): 1057–1064.

9. Jane Duckett, "Political Interests and the Implementation of China's Urban Health Insurance Reform," *Social Policy and Administration* 35, no. 3 (2001): 290–306.

10. Winnie Yip and William Hsiao, "Medical Savings Accounts: Lessons from the People's Republic of China," *Health Affairs* 16, no. 6 (1997): 244–251.

11. Gordon G. Liu, et al., "Equity in Health Care Access: Assessing the Urban Health Insurance Reform in China," *Social Science and Medicine* 55, no. 10 (2002): 1779–1794.

12. *Ibid.*

13. *Ibid.*

14. Xing-zhu Liu and Anne Mills, "Financing Reforms of Public Health Services in China: Lessons for Other Nations," *Social Science and Medicine* 54, no. 11 (2000): 1691- 1698.

15. Duckett, (2001).

16. *Ibid.*

17. *Ibid.*

18. Jun Gao, et al., "Changing Access to Health Services in Urban China: Implications for Equity," *Health Policy and Planning* 16, no. 3 (2001): 302–312.

19. *Ibid.*

20. Gerald Bloom and Xing-yuan Gu, "Health Sector Reform: Lessons from China,"*Social Science and Medicine* 45, no. 3 (2000): 351–360.

21. Hu, (1998).

22. The literature on welfare pluralism is rich. See the following contributions: Neil Gilbert, *Capitalism and the Welfare State* (New Haven, Connecticut: Yale University Press, 1984); Norman Johnson, *The Welfare State in Transition: The Theory and Practice of Welfare Pluralism* (Sussex: Wheatsheaf Books, 1987); Idem., *Reconstructing the Welfare State: A Decade of Change 1980–1990* (Sussex: Wheatsheaf Books, 1990); Idem., ed., *Private Markets in Health and Welfare* (Oxford: Berg Publications, 1995).

23. Hu, (1998).

24. Bitran and Yip, (1998).

25. World Bank, *China: Long-Term Issues and Options in the Health Transition*

(Washington DC: World Bank, 1992); Idem., *Investing in Health: World Development Report* (New York: Oxford University Press, 1993).

26. World Bank, *Financing Health Care: Issues and Options for China* (Washington DC: World Bank, 1997).

27. Joan Kaufman and Fang Jing, "Privatisation of Health Services and the Reproductive Health of Rural Chinese Women," *Reproductive Health Matters* 10, no. 20 (2002): 108–116.

28. Lindert's idea is discussed in chapter 4. His contribution "*Growing Public: Social Spending and Economic Growth since the Eighteenth Century*" (Cambridge: Cambridge University Press, 2004) discusses why advanced countries spend more today on public schools, welfare, public pensions, and redistribution in general than in the past.

29. World Bank, (1997).

30. China entered into the World Trade Organization in 2001.

31. Betty Ho and Thomas Tsai, "The Chairman and the Coronavirus: Globalization and China's Healthcare System," *Harvard International Review* 25, no. 4 (2004): 28–33, 28–29.

32. Duckett, (2001).

33. *Ibid.*, 296.

34. With regard to our recommendation for increased government spending, some encouraging signs are noted. In September 2004, the central government announced its intention to spend some 0.3 billion yuan each year to implement an urban health care aid system. The target groups would include the poor and the vulnerable. The Ministry of Civil Affairs is now drafting the details of the plan. The central government expects this subsidy will be accompanied by a matching fund of the same amount from the local governments. This system was preceded by the one that had been implemented in the rural areas. The initiative came from the new Communist leadership under Party Chairman Hu Jin-tao and Chinese Premier Wen Jia-bao. China Internet Information Center, September 12, 2004, www. china.com.cn (in Chinese).

35. World Health Organization, *The World Health Report 2003—Shaping the Future* (Geneva: WHO, 2003).

36. United Nations, *Human Development Report* 2003 (New York: Oxford

University Press, 2003).

37. Developmentalism is discussed in chapter 4 of the book. On the theory of developmentalism, see the following contributions: James Midgley, "Growth, Redistribution and Welfare: Towards Social Investment," *Social Service Review* 73, no. 1 (1999): 1– 12; Idem., "Globalization, Capitalism and Social Welfare: A Social Development Perspective," *Canadian Social Work Review* 17 (2000): 13–28; Idem., "Poverty and the Social Development Approach," in *Poverty Monitoring and Alleviation in East Asia*, ed. Kwong-leung Tang and Chack-kie Wong (New York: Nova Science Press, 2003), 155–178; James Midgley, Martin Tracy and Michelle Livermore, eds., *The Handbook of Social Policy* (Thousand Oaks, CA: Sage Publications, 2000); James Midgley and Michael Sherraden, "The Social Development Perspective in Social Policy," in *The Handbook of Social Policy*, ed. J. Midgley et al. (Thousand Oaks, CA: Sage Publications, 2000), 435–445; James Midgley and Kwong-leung Tang, "Social Policy, Economic Growth and Developmental Welfare," *International Journal of Social Welfare* 10, no. 4 (2001): 244–252; Kwong-leung Tang, *Social Welfare Development in East Asia* (New York: Palgrave, 2000); and Kwong-leung Tang and Raymond Ngan, "China: Developmentalism and Social Security," *International Journal of Social Welfare* 10, no. 4 (2001): 253–259.

38. Micheal Sherraden, *Assets and the Poor: A New American Welfare Policy*, (New York: M. E. Sharpe,1991).

39. Academics like Duckett argue that the presence of a socially pooled fund preserves some form of collectivism in Communist China. *See* Jane Duckett, "State, Collectivism and Worker Privilege: A Study of Urban Health Insurance Reform," *China Quarterly* 177 (2004): 155–173.

40. Yip and Hsiao, (1996).

41. Bitran and Yip, (1998).

42. Yip and Hsiao, (2001), 23.

43. *Ibid.* WHO, (2003)

44. Duckett, (2001).

45. *Ibid.*, 302.

46. Cheung and Gu, (2004), 49.

47. *See* James Midgley and Kwong-leung Tang, "Social Policy, Economic Growth and Developmental Welfare," *International Journal of Social Welfare 10*, no. 4 (2001): 244–252, and other papers in this special issue on the theory and practice of developmental welfare; Anthony Hall and James Midgley, eds., *Social Policy for Development* (Thousand Oaks, CA: Sage Publications, 2004).

48. Liu and Mills, (2000).

49. James Midgley, *Social Development: The Developmental Perspective in Social Welfare* (Thousand Oaks, CA: Sage Publications, 1995); Idem., *Social Welfare in Global Context* (Thousand Oaks, CA: Sage Publications, 1997).

Appendix

Questionnaire from the Wuhan's Health Care Study 2003[1]

Please ✓in the appropriate ❑

Personal Information

1 Gender

1 ❑ Male 2 ❑ Female

2 How old are you?

_____________________age

3 What is your education level? 9 ❑ Refuse to answer

1 ❑ Illiterate 9 ❑ Refuse to answer

2 ❑ Primary school

3 ❑ Lower secondary

4 ❑ Higher secondary

5 ❑ College

6 ❑ Tertiary or above 1 ❑

4 What is your marital status?

1 ❑ Unmarried 9 ❑ Refuse to answer

2 ❑ Married

3 ❑ Divorced

4 ❑ Remarried (after divorce)

5 ❑ Widowed

6 ❑ Remarried (after loss of spouse)

7 ❑ Other

5 What is the ownership form of your current employment unit?

1 ❑ State owned 9 ❑ Refuse to answer

2 ❑ Collective

3 ❑ Private enterprise/individual ownership

4 ❑ Joint venture/securitized enterprises[2]

5 ❑ Foreign/Hong Kong/Taiwan and Macau investment

6 ❑ Other

6 What is the average monthly income of your principal employment?

01 ❑ Below ¥300
02 ❑ ¥300–¥499
03 ❑ ¥500–¥999
04 ❑ ¥1,000–¥1,499
05 ❑ ¥1,500–¥1,999
06 ❑ ¥2,000–¥2,499
07 ❑ ¥2,500–¥2,999
08 ❑ ¥3,000–¥3,999
09 ❑ ¥4,000–¥4,999
10 ❑ ¥5,000–¥7,499
11 ❑ ¥7,500–¥9,999
12 ❑ ¥10,000 or above
99 ❑ Refuse to answer

7 What is the nature of your present post: a permanent worker, a contracted worker, or a temporary worker?

1 ❑ Permanent
2 ❑ Contracted
3 ❑ Temporary
9 ❑ Refuse to answer

(Location in the original questionnaire: Q1, Q2, Q4, Q5, Q7, Q11, and Q8)

Questions for Table 5.2:
Experiences with using medial insurance

2.1 Do you have experience using your personal account for paying medical expenses?

1 ❑ Have
2 ❑ Have not
8 ❑ Not applicable
9 ❑ Refuse to answer

2.2 Do you have experience using the social insurance fund for paying medical expenses?

1 ❑ Have
2 ❑ Have not
8 ❑ Not applicable
9 ❑ Refuse to answer

2.3 Do you have experience claiming insurance beyond the ceiling of the social insurance fund due to serious illness?

1 ❑ Have
2 ❑ Have not
8 ❑ Not applicable
9 ❑ Refuse to answer

(Location in the original questionnaire: Q28, Q30, and Q31)

Questions for Table 5.3:
Participation in supplemental health insurance

3.1 Have labor unions or other organizations organized some voluntary supplemental insurance schemes?

1 ❑ Yes
2 ❑ No
9 ❑ Refuse to answer

3.2 Have you purchased commercial medical insurance?

1 ❑ Have
2 ❑ Have not
9 ❑ Refuse to answer

(Location in the original questionnaire: Q18 and Q19)

Questions for Table 5.4:
Features of Basic Health Insurance

4.1 Do you agree that the current arrangement of the social insurance fund and a personal account is reasonable?

1 ❑ Strongly disagree
2 ❑ Disagree
3 ❑ Half-half
4 ❑ Agree
5 ❑ Strongly agree
8 ❑ Don't know/no idea
9 ❑ Refuse to answer

4.2 Which fund, the social insurance fund or the personal account, should be allocated more?

1 ❑ Strongly disagree
2 ❑ Disagree
8 ❑ Don't know/no idea
9 ❑ Refuse to answer

4.3 Do you agree that it is reasonable for an individual to bear part of his or her medical expenses?

1 ❑ Strongly disagree
2 ❑ Disagree
3 ❑ Half-half
4 ❑ Agree
5 ❑ Strongly agree
8 ❑ Don't know/no idea
9 ❑ Refuse to answer

(Location in the original questionnaire: Q36, Q37, and Q43c)

Questions for Table 5.5:
Effects of reform initiatives on hospitals

How far do you agree with the following statement about health care reform?

	1	2	3	4	5	8	9
5.1 Health care reforms can reduce patient's abuse of health service, such as treating minor illness as serious illness	❑	❑	❑	❑	❑	❑	❑
5.2 Health care reform can reduce doctor's intentional prescription of expensive drugs	❑	❑	❑	❑	❑	❑	❑
5.3 Now consulting doctors is more convenient than it was before	❑	❑	❑	❑	❑	❑	❑
5.4 Now patients have more choices of doctors and hospitals than they had before	❑	❑	❑	❑	❑	❑	❑
5.5 Now service quality provided by doctors and hospitals is better than it was before	❑	❑	❑	❑	❑	❑	❑

[5-point scale with 1=strongly disagree; 2=disagree; 3=half-half; 4=agree; 5=strongly agree; 8=don't know/no idea; and 9=refuse to answer]
(Location in the original questionnaire: Q33e, Q33f, Q33g, Q33h, andQ33j)

Questions for Table 5.6:
Control of the costs of medicine

6.1 Do you agree that the current limit on reimbursement of medicine is reasonable?

1 ❑ Strongly disagree
2 ❑ Disagree
3 ❑ Half-half
4 ❑ Agree
5 ❑ Strongly agree
8 ❑ Don't know/no idea
9 ❑ Refuse to answer

6.2 How do you feel about the proportion of drug cost to medical consultation?

1 ❑ Very high
2 ❑ High
3 ❑ Average
4 ❑ Low
5 ❑ Very low
6 ❑ Forgotten
9 ❑ Refuse to answer

6.3 Where is the most cost-effective place to purchase drugs?

1 ❑ Hospitals/clinics
2 ❑ Pharmacies
3 ❑ Units' clinics
4 ❑ Other
9 ❑ Refuse to answer

6.4 Where is the usual place to purchase drugs after medical consultation in hospitals and clinics?

1 ❑ Hospitals/clinics
2 ❑ Pharmacies
3 ❑ Units' clinics
4 ❑ Other
9 ❑ Refuse to answer

(Location in the original questionnaire: Q33i, Q25, Q27, and Q26)

Questions for Table 5.7:
Responsibility in health care

How far do you agree with the following statements about responsibility in health care?

	1	2	3	4	5	8	9
7.1 Those who are not able to pay for medical fees should be assisted by the government or the employment unit	❑	❑	❑	❑	❑	❑	❑
7.2 The government has no responsibility to provide basic health care to all	❑	❑	❑	❑	❑	❑	❑

7.3 It is reasonable to treat urban and rural residents differently in terms of health care benefits	☐	☐	☐	☐	☐	☐	☐
7.4 One should not be entitled to health care protection if one does not pay for medical insurance	☐	☐	☐	☐	☐	☐	☐

[5-point scale with 1=strongly disagree; 2=disagree; 3=half-half; 4=agree; 5=strongly agree; 8=don't know/no idea; and 9=refuse to answer]

7.5 Are medical expenses the primary responsibility of individuals, employment units, or the government?

1 ☐ Individuals
2 ☐ Employment units
3 ☐ Government
8 ☐ Don't know/no idea
9 ☐ Refuse to answer

7.6 Which one of the following should be responsible for medical expenses above the ceiling if patients do not have medical insurance for serious illness?

1 ☐ Patients and their families
2 ☐ Patients' employment units
3 ☐ Government
8 ☐ Don't know/no idea
9 ☐ Refuse to answer

(Location in the original questionnaire: Q43j, Q29a, Q29c, Q29d, Q42, and Q32)

Questions for Table 5.8:
Out-of-pocket payment for health care

How far do you agree with the following statement about out-of-pocket payment for health care?

	1	2	3	4	5	8	9
8.1 Out-of-pocket payment for expert consultation is right	☐	☐	☐	☐	☐	☐	☐
8.2 Out-of-pocket payment for high-tech medical equipment is right	☐	☐	☐	☐	☐	☐	☐
8.3 Out-of-pocket payment for high-quality medicines is right	☐	☐	☐	☐	☐	☐	☐
8.4 Out-of-pocket payment for staying at high-class wards is right	☐	☐	☐	☐	☐	☐	☐

[5-point scale with 1=strongly disagree; 2=disagree; 3=half-half; 4=agree; 5=strongly agree; 8=don't know/no idea; and 9=refuse to answer]
(Location in the original questionnaire: Q43f, Q43g, Q43h, and Q43i)

Questions for Table 5.9:
Economic development and health care

How far do you agree with the following statement about economic development and health care?

	1	2	3	4	5	8	9
9.1 The primary role of the government is economic development and not welfare improvement	❑	❑	❑	❑	❑	❑	❑
9.2 Medical expenses exceed what our country can afford under the current economic condition	❑	❑	❑	❑	❑	❑	❑
9.3 The current medical examination and treatment expenses exceed what the general public can afford	❑	❑	❑	❑	❑	❑	❑

[5-point scale with 1=strongly disagree; 2=disagree; 3=half-half; 4=agree; 5=strongly agree; 8=don't know/no idea; and 9=refuse to answer]
(Location in the original questionnaire: Q43b, Q29e, and Q29f)

Questions for Table 5.10:
Overall outcome of health care reform

How far do you agree with the following statement about overall outcome of health care reform?

	1	2	3	4	5	8	9
10.1 The health care system must be changed	❑	❑	❑	❑	❑	❑	❑
10.2 The current health care protection in Wuhan is better than that before the economic reform	❑	❑	❑	❑	❑	❑	❑
10.4 It is common that people are afraid of seeking medical consultation when they are ill in Wuhan	❑	❑	❑	❑	❑	❑	❑
10.7 I don't worry about Wuhan's future health care protection	❑	❑	❑	❑	❑	❑	❑

[5-point scale with 1=strongly disagree; 2=disagree; 3=half-half; 4=agree; 5=strongly agree; 8=don't know/no idea; and 9=refuse to answer]

10.3 How do you feel about the current individual responsibility of medical expenses?

1 ❑ Too heavy
2 ❑ Just fine
3 ❑ Can bear more
8 ❑ Don't know/no idea
9 ❑ Refuse to answer

10.5 Do you worry about medical expenses in the case of serious illness?

1 ❑ Worry a lot
2 ❑ Worry
3 ❑ Half-half
4 ❑ Not worry
5 ❑ Completely not worry
8 ❑ Don't know/no idea
9 ❑ Refuse to answer

10.6 Do you worry about health care protection after retirement?

1 ❑ Worry a lot
2 ❑ Worry
3 ❑ Half-half
4 ❑ Not worry
5 ❑ Completely not worry
8 ❑ Don't know/no idea
9 ❑ Refuse to answer

(Location in the original questionnaire: Q33d, Q33c, Q33a, Q33b, Q39, Q41, and Q40)

Notes

1. We have two questionnaires: one for employees and one for patients. Except for a few questions, all are the same. Only the selected questions for the tables in chapter 5 are presented here.
2. Enterprises with stocks owned by non-state owners.

Bibliography

Andersen, J. G. "Health Care in the People's Republic of China: A Blend of Traditional and Modern." *Central Issues in Anthropology* 10 (1992): 67–75.

Bai Jian-feng. "What Does Medical Reform Bring?" *Renmin Ribao*, 12 January 2001. (in Chinese).

Beck, Paul A., Hal G. Rainery, Keith Nichols, and Carol Traut. "Disadvantage, Disaffection, and Race as Divergent Bases for Citizen Fiscal Policy Preferences." *Journal of Politics* 52, no. 1 (February 1990): 71–93.

Beijing Qingnianbao. "The Latest Statistics of the Ministry of Health: The Average Cost of a Doctor Visit Is 79 Yuan." 18 August 2000 (in Chinese).

Benatar, Solomon R., Abdallah Daar, and Peter Singer. "Global Health Ethics: The Rationale for Mutual Caring." *International Affair* 79, no. 1 (2003): 107–138.

Beveridge, William. *Social Insurance and Allied Services*. London: HMSO, 1942.

Bhatia, Mrigesh, and Elias Mossialos. "Health Systems in Developing Countries." In *Social Policy for Development*, edited by A. Hall and J. Midgley, 168–204. Thousand Oaks, Calfornia: Sage Publications, 2004.

Bitran, Ricardo, and Winnie C. Yip. "A Review of Health Care Provider Payment Reform in Selected Countries in Asia and Latin America." Major Applied Research 2, Working Paper 1. Bethesda, Maryland: Partnerships for Health Reform Project, Abt Associates, August 1998.

Bloom, Gerald, and Xing-yuan Gu. "Health Sector Reform: Lessons from China." *Social Science and Medicine* 45, no. 3 (2000): 351–360.

Briggs, Asa. "The Welfare State in Historical Perspective." *Europene de Sociologie* 2, no. 2 (1961): 212–258.

Castano, Ramon A., Jose J. Arbelaez, Ursula B. Giedion, and Luis G..Morales. "Equitable Financing, Out-of-Pocket Payments and the Role of Health Care Reform in Colombia." *Health Policy and Planning* 17, no. 1 (2002): S5–S11.

Chen, Jia-gui and Yan-zhong Wang. "The Report on China's Urban Health Care System." in *China Social Security System Development Report 1997–2001*, edited by Jia-gui Chen, 76–113. Beijing: Shehui Kexue Wenxian Chubanshe, 2001 (in Chinese).

Cheung, Anthony, and Xing-yuan Gu. "Health Finance." In *Social Policy Reform in Hong Kong and Shanghai: A Tale of Two Cities*, edited by Linda Wong, Lynn White, and Shixun Gui, 23–52. Armonk, NY: M. E. Sharpe, 2004.

China Information News, "*Xiaokang*: People are Searching for a Hundred Methods." 4 December 2002. Downloaded from www.people.com.cn. 4 August 2003 (in Chinese).

China Information News, "National Statistical Bureau Forecast: Three-fourths of People Enter *Xiaokang* This Year End." 23 November 2003. Downloaded from www.people.com.cn. 4 August 2003 (in Chinese).

China National Statistical Bureau. *Statistical Bulletin on National Economic and Social Development 2003*. Downloaded from www.stats.gov.cn/tjgb/ndtjgb/qgndtjgb/t20040226_402131958.htm (in Chinese).

The Chinese Communist Party. *The Resolution of the 3rd Plenary of the 16th Party Congress*, Downloaded from www.people.com.cn. 14 October 2003 (in Chinese).

Colclough, Christopher. ed. *Marketizing Education and Health in Developing Countries*. Oxford: Clarendon, 1997.

Cook, Sarah, and Gordon White. "Alternative Approaches to Welfare Policy Analysis: New Institutional Economics, Politics, and Political Economy." In *Social Provisions in Low-Income Countries: New Patterns and Emerging Trends*, edited by Germano Mwabu, Cecilia Ugaz, and Gordon White, 26–52. Oxford: Oxford University Press, 2001.

Dai, Lu-guo. "The Guarantee of Medical Care Is Not a Dream." *China Labor* 182 (February 2001): 4–6 (in Chinese).

Development Research Center of the State Council. "The Comparison of China with Countries at US$3,000 GDP per capita." Downloaded from www.drcnet.com.cn. 4 May 2004 (in Chinese).

Ding, Wei."Documentary Facts about Shanghai's Reform of the Health System." *Renmin Ribao*. 28 August 2000 (in Chinese).

Dixon, John, and Mark Hyde, eds. *The Marketization of Social Security: International Perspectives*. Westport, CT: Quorum Books, 2001.

Dorn, James A., ed. *China in the New Millennium*. Washington DC: Cato Institute, 1998.

Duckett, Jane. "Political Interests and the Implementation of China's Urban Health Insurance Reform." *Social Policy and Administration* 35, no. 3 (2001): 290–306.

——."State, Collectivism and Worker Privilege: A Study of Urban Health Insurance Reform." *China Quarterly* 177 (2004): 155–173.

Esping-Andersen, Gosta, with Duncan Gallic, Anton Hemerijck and John Myles. *Why We Need A New Welfare State*. Thousand Oaks, CA: Sage Publication, 2002.

Field, Mark G., ed. *Success and Crisis in National Health Systems: A Comparative Approach*. New York: Routledge, 1989.

Flood, Colleen, M. *International Health Care Reform: A Legal, Economic and Political Analysis*. London and New York: Routledge, 2000.

Gao, Jun, Sheng-lan Tang, Rachel Tolhurst, and Ke-qing Rao. "Changing Access to Health Services in Urban China: Implications for Equity." *Health Policy and Planning* 16, no. 3 (2001): 302–312.

Gao. Jun, Jun-cheng Qian, Sheng-lan Tang, Bo Eriksson, and Erik Blas. "Health Equity in Transition from Planned to Market Economy in China." *Health Policy and Planning* 17, no. 1 (2002): S20–S29.

Giaimo, Susan, and Philip Manow. "Adapting the Welfare State." *Comparative Political Studies* 32, no. 8 (1999): 967–1000.

Gilbert, Neil. *Capitalism and the Welfare State*. New Haven, CT: Yale University Press, 1984.

Gong, Sen. "China's Financial Health Input and the Analysis of its Performance since Economic Reform." Internal report no. 2, Social Development Department, Development Research Center, State Council, August 2004.

Griffin, Charles C. *Health Care in Asia: A Comparative Study of Cost and Financing*. Washington DC: World Bank, 1992.
Grogan, Colleen M. "Urban Economic Reform and Access to Health Care Coverage in the People's Republic of China." *Social Science and Medicine* 41, no. 8 (1995): 1073–84.
Guan, Xin-ping, "Poverty and Antipoverty Policies in Urban China." In *Poverty Monitoring and Alleviation in East Asia*, edited by Kwong-leung Tang and Chack-kie Wong, 15–37. New York: Nova science Press, 2003.
Guo, Bao-gang. "Transforming China's Urban Health System." *Asian Survey* 43, no. 2 (March/April 2003): 385–403.
Hadley, Roger, and Stephen Hatch. *Social Welfare and the Failure of the State*. London: Allen and Unwin, 1981.
Hall, Anthony, and James Midgley, eds. *Social Policy for Development*. Thousand Oaks, CA: Sage Publications, 2004.
Ho, Betty, and Thomas Tsai. "The Chairman and the Coronavirus: Globalization and China's Healthcare System." *Harvard International Review* 25, no. 4 (2004): 28–31.
Hospital Authority. "*Annual Report of Hospital Authority, 2002–2003*." Downloaded from www.ha.org.hk. 17 January 2004.
Hsia Po-guang. "Enthusiastic Discussion of Medical Care Protection by Representatives." *China Social Security System* 4 (2003): 20–23 (in Chinese).
Hsiao, William, C. L. "The Chinese Health Care System: Lessons for Other Nations." *Social Science and Medicine* 41, no. 8 (1995): 1047–1055.
Hu, The-wai, and Chee-ruey Hsieh. *The Economics of Health Care in Asia-Pacific Countries*. Cheltenham: Edward Edgar, 2002.
Hu, Zu-liu. "Social Protection and Enterprise Reform." In *Enterprise and Social Benefits from Communism*, edited by M. Rein, B. Friedman and A. Worgotter, 284–304. Cambridge University Press: Cambridge, 1998.
Hyde, Mark, and John Dixon. "Welfare Ideology, the Market and Security: Toward a Typology of Market-Oriented Reform." In *The Marketization of Social Security*, edited by M. Hyde and J. Dixon, 51–80. Westport, CT: Quorum, 2001.
Janes, Craig R. "The Health Transition, Global Modernity and the Crisis of Traditional Medicine: The Tibetan Case." *Social Science and Medicine* 48 (1999): 1803–1820.
Johnson, Norman. *The Welfare State in Transition: The Theory and Practice of Welfare Pluralism*. Sussex: Wheatsheaf Books, 1987.
——.*Reconstructing the Welfare State: A Decade of Change 1980–1990*. Sussex: Wheatsheaf Books, 1990.
——,ed. *Private Markets in Health and Welfare*. Oxford: Berg Publications, 1995.
Kamerman, Sheila B., and Alfred J. Kahn, eds. *Privatization and the Welfare State*. Princeton, NJ: Princeton University Press, 1989.
Kangas, Olli E. "Self Interest and the Common Good: the Impact of Norms, Selfishness and Context in Social Policy Opinions." *Journal of Socio-Economics* 26, no. 5 (1997): 475–494.
Kaufman, Joan, and Fang Jing. "Privatisation of Health Services and the Reproductive Health of Rural Chinese Women." *Reproductive Health Matters* 10, no. 20 (2002): 108–116.
Lahelma, Eero, Katariina Kivelä, Eva Roos, Terhi Tuominen, Espen Dahl, Finn Diderichsen, Jon Ivar Elstad, Inge Lissau, Olle Lundberg, Ossi Rahkonen, Niels Kristian Rasmussen, and Monica Åberg Yngwe. "Analysing Changes of Health

Inequalities in the Nordic Welfare States." *Social Science and Medicine* 55 (2002): 609–625.

Lassey, Marie L., William R. Lassey, and Martin J. Jinks. *Health Care Systems Around the World: Characteristics, Issues and Reforms*. New Jersey: Prentice Hall, 1997. Leung, Joe C.B., and Richard C. Nann. *Authority and Benevolence, Social Welfare in China*. Hong Kong: The Chinese University Press, 1995. Lewis, Jane. *The Voluntary Sector, the State and Social Work*. Aldershot: Edward Elgar, 1995.

Li, Lan-qing. Speech at the National Conference on the Reforms of the Basic Health Insurance System and the Health and Medicine System for Urban Staff and Workers. 24–26 July 2000 (in Chinese).

Li, Pei-lin. "Problems and Trends of China's Social and Economic Developments." Article form *China.com*. Downloaded from http://china.com.cn/chinese/zhuanti/2004shxs/483054.htm. 17 January 2004 (in Chinese).

Li, Tong-xin. "What Are the Difficulties in Controlling Drug Prices?" *Shichangbao*, 29 June 2000 (in Chinese).

Lindert, Peter H. *Growing Public: Social Spending and Economic Growth since the Eighteenth Century*. Cambridge: Cambridge University Press, 2004.

Liu, Gordon G., Ren-hua Cai, Zhong-yun Zhao, Peter Yuen, Xian-jun Xiong, Shumarry Chao, and Bo-qing Wang. "Urban Health Care Reform Initiative in China: Findings from its Pilot Experiment in Zhengjiang City." *International Journal of Economic Development* 4 (1999): 504–526.

Liu, Gordon G., Zhong-yun Zhao, Ren-hua Cai, Tetsuji Yamada and Tadashi Yamada. "Equity in Health Care Access: Assessing the Urban Health Insurance Reform in China." *Social Science and Medicine* 55, no. 10 (2002): 1779–1794.

Liu, Shu-duo. "How to Change in the Reform of Hospitals?" *China Economic Times*, 24 March 2004. Downloaded from http://news.sohu.com (in Chinese).

Liu, Xing-zhu, and J. L. Wang. "An Introduction to China's Health Care System." *Journal of Public Health Policy* 2, no. 1 (1991): 104–116.

Liu, Xing-zhu and William Hsiao. "The Cost Escalation of Social Health Insurance Plans in China: Its Implication for Public Policy." *Social Science and Medicine* 41, no.8 (1995): 1095–1101.

Liu, Xing-zhu, and Anne Mills. "Financing Reforms of Public Health Services in China: Lessons for Other Nations." *Social Science and Medicine* 54, no. 11 (2000): 1691–1698.

Liu, Yuan-li, William C. Hsiao, and Karen Eggleston. "Equity in Health and Health Care: the Chinese Experience." *Social Science and Medicine* 49, no. 10 (1999): 1349–1356.

Liu, Zhong-xian. "A Study of the Problem Related to Medical Assistance for Urban Poor."

Unpublished manuscript, Sociology Department, the People's University of China, 2003 (In Chinese).

Martin, Michael, and Jane Sell. "The Role of the Experiment in the Social Sciences." *The Sociological Quarterly* 20, no. 4 (1979): 581–590.

Midgley, James. *Social Development: The Developmental Perspective in Social Welfare*. Thousand Oaks, CA: Sage Publications, 1995.

——.*Social Welfare in Global Context*. Thousand Oaks, CA: Sage Publications, 1997.

——."Growth, Redistribution and Welfare: Towards Social Investment." *Social Service Review* 73. no. 1 (1999): 1–12.

——."Globalization, Capitalism and Social Welfare: A Social Development Perspective." Special issue, *Canadian Social Work Review* 17 (July 2000): 13–28.

——."Poverty and the Social Development Approach." In *Poverty Monitoring and Alleviation in East Asia*, edited by Kwong-leung Tang and Chack-kie Wong, 155–178. New York: Nova Science Press, 2003.

Midgley, James, Martin Tracy and Michelle Livermore, eds. *The Handbook of Social Policy*. Thousand Oaks, CA: Sage Publications, 2000.

Midgley, James, and Michael Sherraden. "The Social Development Perspective in Social Policy." In *The Handbook of Social Policy*, edited by James Midgley, Martin B. Tracy and Michelle Livermore, 435–445. Thousand Oaks, CA: Sage Publications, 2000.

Midgley, James, and Kwong-leung Tang. "Social Policy, Economic Growth and Developmental Welfare." *International Journal of Social Welfare* 10, no. 4 (2001): 244–252.

Ministry of Health, *An Analysis Report of the Second National Health Survey, 1998*. (July 1999). Downloaded from www.moh.gov.cn/statistics/ronhs98/ ronhus4/.doc 4 May 2004 (in Chinese).

——.*Brief Report of the Development of Health Affairs in China, 1997–2001*. Downloaded from www.moh.gov.cn/tjxxzx/tjsj/tjgb/1200304030003.htm. 23 January 2003 (in Chinese).

——.*Summary of China's Health Statistics, 2004*. Downloaded from www.moh.gov.cn/statistics. 4 May 2004 (in Chinese).

——."Notice Concerning the Management of Consultation Items of City and Township Employee under Basic Medical Insurance." no. 44 (30 June 1999) (in Chinese).

Ministry of Labor and Social Security. "Notice Concerning the Temporary Control in the Use of Drugs of City and Township Employees under Basic Medical Insurance." no. 15 (12 May 1999) (in Chinese).

Mishra, Ramesh. *Society and Social Policy*. London: Macmillan, 1981.

——.*The Welfare State in Crisis*. Brighton: Wheatsheaf Books, 1984.

Mwabu, Germano, Cecilia Ugaz, and Gordon White, eds. *Social Provisions in Low-Income Countries: New Patterns and Emerging Trends*. Oxford: Oxford University Press, 2001.

Mwabu, Germano, Reino Hjerppe, Cecilia Ugaz, and Gordon White. "Introduction: Context and Scope." In *Social Provisions in Low-Income Countries: New Patterns and Emerging Trends*, edited by G. Mwabu, C. Ugaz, G. White. Oxford: Oxford University Press, 2001.

National Bureau of Statistics of China. *China Statistical Yearbook 2003*. Beijing: China Statistics Press, 2003 (in Chinese).

Newbrander, William, and Patricia Moser. "Private Health Sector Growth in Asia: An Introduction." In *Private Health Sector Growth in Asia*, edited by W. Newbrander, 1- 10. Chichester: John Wiley and Sons, 1997a.

——."The Future of Health Sector Reform in Asia." In *Private Health Sector Growth in Asia*, edited by W. Newbrander, 221–229. Chichester: John Wiley and Sons, 1997b.

Payne, Malcolm. *Modern Social Work Theory*. Chicago; Lyceum Books, 1997.

Pei, Xiao-mei, and Vijiyan K. Pillai. "Old Age Support in China: The Role of the State and the Family." *International Journal of Aging and Human Development* 49, no. 3 (1999): 197–212.

Peng, Pei-yun. "Opening Speech at the National Conference on the Expansion of Trial Work for the Reform of Health Care System for Staff and Workers, 8 April 1996."

in *The Reform of the Health Care System for Staff and Workers*, edited by Distribution and Social Security Department of the State Structural Reform Commission, et al., 3–21. Beijing: Gaige Chubanshe, 1996 (in Chinese).

Pierson, Christopher. *Beyond the Welfare State*. Cambridge: Polity, 1991.

Pinker, Robert. *Social Theory and Social Policy*. London: Heinemann, 1979.

——."Making Sense of the Mixed Economy of Welfare." *Social Policy and Administration* 26, no. 4 (1992): 273–284.

Powell, Martin, and Martin Hewitt, *Welfare State and Welfare Change*. Buckingham; Philadelphia: Open University Press, 2002.

Romanow, R.J. *Building on Values: The Future of Health Care in Canada 2002*. Downloaded from www.healthcarecommission.ca/default.asp?DN=cn=2,ou=Stories, ou=Suite247,o=HCC. 17 January 2003.

Sen, Amartya. *Development as Freedom*. NY: Anchor Books, 1999.

Sherraden, Michael. *Assets and the Poor: A New American Welfare Policy*. Armonk, NY: M.E. Sharpe, 1991.

Smyth, Russell. "Labor-Market and Social-Welfare Reform in the State-Owned Sector in China." *Journal of Developing Areas* 33, no. 2 (1999): 223–244.

Social Security Research Institute. "An Investigative and Analytical Report on the Reform of the Health Insurance Systems in Zhenjiang, Changshu, and Shanghai." Unpublished report, the Ministry of Labor and Social Security of the People's Republic of China, 11 November 2001.

Social Policy Research Center, China Academy of Social Science. *An Overview of Rural Health Care Protection*, (Unpublished report, March 2003).

Song, Xiao-wu, and Hao Liu. "The Reform of the Health Insurance System and Accompanying Measures" in *Report on the Reform and Development of China's Social Security System*, edited by Xiao-wu Song. Beijing: The Renmin University of China Chubanshe, 2001 (in Chinese), 83–106.

Spicker, Stuart F. "Going Off the Dole: A Prudential and Ethical Critique of the 'Healthfare' State." In *Reforming Health Care: The Philosophy and Practice of International Health Reform*, edited by David Seedhouse, 131–142. Chicester: John Wiley and Sons, 1995.

Starr, Paul. "The Meaning of Privatization." In *Privatization and the Welfare State*, edited by S. Kamerman and A. Kahn, 15–48. Princeton, NJ: Princeton University Press, 1989.

——."The Limits of Privatization." In *Privatization and Deregulation in Global Perspective*, edited by D. J. Gayle and J. N. Goodrich, 109–125. New York: Quorum Books, 1990.

Statistics and Information Center, Ministry of Health. An *Analysis Report of the Second National Health Survey*, 1998. Downloaded from www.moh.gov.cn/statistics/ronhs98/ronhs41.doc. 7 July 2004.

Tang, Kwong-leung. "The Case for the Privatization of Social Welfare: Three Decades of Public Opinion from Great Britain and the United States." *Scandinavian Journal of Social Welfare* no. 6 (1997): 34–43.

——.*Social Welfare Development in East Asia*. New York: Palgrave, 2000.

Tang, Kwong-leung, and Raymond Ngan. "China: Developmentalism and Social Security." *International Journal of Social Welfare 10*, no. 4 (2001): 253–259.

Tang, Kwong-leung, and James Midgley. "Social Policy after the East Asian Crisis: Forging a Normative Basis for Welfare." *Journal of Asian Comparative*

Development 1, no. 2 (2002): 301–318.

Tanner, Michael. "Using Market Mechanisms to Provide Retirement Security and Health Care in China." In *China in the New Millennium: Market Reforms and Social Development*, edited by James A. Dorn, 319-330. Washington DC: Cato Institute, 1998.

The Economist. Special Report: China's Health Care. 21 August 2004, 20–22.

Titmuss, Richard. *Social Policy*. London: Unwin Hyman, 1974.

Twaddle, Andrew C. "Health System Reforms: Toward a Framework for International Comparisons." *Social Science and Medicine* 43, no. 5 (1996): 637–654.

United Nations. *Human Development Report 2003*. New York: Oxford University Press, 2003.

van de Ven, Wynand P.M.M. "Market-oriented Health Care Reforms: Trends and Future Options." *Social Science and Medicine* 43, no. 5 (1996): 655–666.

——."Equity, Cost Containment and Efficiency in Health Care: Can They Be Achieved by Regulated Competition?" In *Ageing, Social Security and Affordability*, edited by Theodore R. Marmor, and Philip R. De Jong, Brookfield, VT: Ashgate, 1998.

Walker, Alan. *Social Planning: A Strategy for Socialist Welfare*. Oxford: Basil Blackwell, 1984.

Wang, Dong-jin. "The Importance and Urgency of Sufficiently Understanding the Reform of the Health Insurance System for Urban Staff and Workers." *China Labor* 158 (January 1999): 4–7 (in Chinese).

——,ed. *The Reform and Development of China's Social Security System*, 278–79. Beijing: Falu Chubanshe, 2001 (in Chinese).

Wang, Hong, and Chun-guang Wang. "Some Thoughts about Building the Basic Medical Protection System for the Poor People in City and Towns." *Labor Protection World* no. 2 (2003): 18–20 (In Chinese).

Wang, Shao-gang. "The Crisis and Change of the Chinese Public Health." *Comparative Studies* (July 2003): 52–88.

Watts, Jonathan. "China's Shift in HIV/AIDS Policy Marks Turnaround on Health," *The Lancet* 363, no. 9418 (April 2004): 1370–1371.

White, Gordon. "Social Security Reforms in China: Toward an East Asian Model?" In *The East Asian Welfare Model*, edited by R. Goodman, G. White and Huck-ju Kwon, 175–198. New York: Routledge, 1998.

Wong, Chack-kie. "Reforming China's State Socialist Workfare System: A Cautionary and Incremental Approach." *Issues and Studies* 35, no. 5 (September/October 1999): 169–194.

Wong, Chack-kie, and Nan-shong P. Li. "Popular Belief in State Intervention for Social Protection in China." *Journal of Social Policy* 29, no. 1 (2000): 109–116.

World Bank. *Financing Health Services in Developing Countries: An Agenda for Reform*. Washington DC: Author, 1987.

——.*China: Long-Term Issues and Options in the Health Transition*, Washington D.C.: World Bank. 1992.

——.*Investing in Health: World Development Report*. New York: Oxford University Press, 1993.

——.*China: Issues and Options in Health Financing*. Washington DC: World Bank, 1996.

——.*Financing Health Care: Issues and Options for China*. China 2020 Series. Washington DC: World Bank, 1997.

World Health Organization. *Evaluation of the Strategy for Health for All by the Year 2000: Seventh Report on the World Health Situation.* Geneva: WHO, Regional Office for the West Pacific, 1987.

——.World Health Report 2000—*Health System: Improving Performance.* Geneva: WHO, 2000. Downloaded from www.who.int/whr2001/2001/archives/2000/en/index.htm. 7 August 2004.

——.*The World Health Report 2003—Shaping the Future.* Geneva: WHO, 2003.

Wu, Ritu. "Establishing and Perfecting a System of Multi-Layered Health Insurance." *China Labor* 163 (June 1999): 11–12 (in Chinese).

Wuhan Municipal Government. "The City Conditions of Wuhan." Downloaded from www.whtj.gov.cn/whsq/whsq2004/index.htm. 5 September 2004 (in Chinese).

Wuhan Statistical Bureau. "Statistical Release of 2003 National Economic and Social Development of Wuhan City." Downloaded from www.whtj.gov.cn/tjgb/2003NGB.htm. 23 February 2004 (in Chinese).

——.*Wuhan Statistical Yearbook,* 2003. Downloaded from www.whtj.gov.cn/whtjnj/tjnj2003/zy/index.htm. 23 April 2004 (in Chinese).

Yan, Hua. "China Debates Medical Reform Privatization." Downloaded from www.atimes.com/atimes/China/FH11Ad04.html. 26 August 2004.

Yang, Pel-lin, Vivian Lin, and James Lawson. "Health Policy Reform in the People's Republic of China." *International Journal of Health Services* 21, no. 3 (1991): 481–491.

Yip, Winnie, and William Hsiao, "Medical Savings Accounts: Lessons from the People's Republic of China." *Health Affairs* 16, no. 6 (1997): 244–251.

Yu, Dei-zhi. "Market-Based Reforms and Changes in China's Health Care System." In *Social Provisions in Low-Income Countries: New Patterns and Emerging Trends,* edited by G. Mwabu, C. Ugaz, and G. White, 265–287. Oxford: Oxford University Press, 2001.

Yu, Wei. "The Important Issue of Enterprise Reform: Health Care Insurance System" in *The Reformability of China's State Sector,* edited by Guan-zhong J. Wen and Dian-qing Xu, 433–63. Singapore: World Scientific Publishing Co., 1997.

Yu, Zi-you, Jin-liang Mo, and Long-xing Wang. "Health Care Expenses and Reform in China." *WCCS Papers* 7, no. 2 (March 1997): 1–14.

Zhang, Fan. "Behind the Desolation of Designated Pharmacies under Health Insurance" *China Economic Times,* 24 March 2004. Downloaded from http://news.sohu.com. (in Chinese).

Zheng Xiang, and Sheila Hillier, "The Reforms of the Chinese Health Care System: County Level Changes: The Jiangxi Study." *Social Science and Medicine* 41, no. 8 (1995): 1057–1064.

Zhenjiang Medical Insurance Bureau. "Zhenjiang Health Care Reform." Downloaded from www.zjyb.gov.cn/ybjj/htm. 6 September 2002 (in Chinese).

——."A General Account of Health Care Reform" Downloaded from www.zjyb.gov.cn/ybjj/htm. 24 August 2004 (in Chinese).

Zhuan, Hui-lin. "Urban Deprived Groups in the New Era: Studying the Construction of a Health Care Protection Mechanism." *Market and Population Analysis* (23 May 2003): 23–28 (in Chinese).

Index

About the Authors

Chack-Kie Wong is a professor at the Department of Social Work, the Chinese University of Hong Kong. His academic interests include comparative social policy, welfare attitudes, and Chinese social welfare. He has published various articles in social policy journals and is the co-editor of the books *East Asian Welfare Regimes in Transition* (Policy Press, Bristol, 2005) and *Poverty Monitoring and Alleviation in East Asia* (Nova, New York, 2003).

Vai Io Lo specializes in Asian and comparative law, especially American, Chinese, and Japanese laws. Currently, she is teaching at the International University of Japan. She is the author of various articles in law journals and the books *Law and Industrial Relations: China and Japan after World War II* (Kluwer, London, 1999) and *Law and Investment in China: The Legal and Business Environments after WTO Accession* (Routledge, London, 2004) (Co-author: Tian, Xiaowen).

Kwong-leung Tang is Chair and Professor of Social Work at the Department of Social Work, the Chinese University of Hong Kong. He is the author of *Social Welfare Development in East Asia* (Macmillan & St. Martin's Press, New York, 2000) and a co-editor of the two volume set entitled *What is Globalization? Critical Perspectives from North and South* and *What is Globalization? Critical Regional Perspectives* (Palgrave, New York, forthcoming). His academic interests include East Asian social welfare, law and social policy, and human rights.

www.ingramcontent.com/pod-product-compliance
Ingram Content Group UK Ltd.
Pitfield, Milton Keynes, MK11 3LW, UK
UKHW041123071026
15587UKWH00009B/128

9 780739 106600